Fire and Rescue Services

Peter Murphy • Kirsten Greenhalgh
Editors

Fire and Rescue Services

Leadership and Management Perspectives

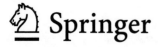 Springer

Editors
Peter Murphy
Nottingham Business School
Nottingham Trent University
Nottingham, UK

Kirsten Greenhalgh
Nottingham University Business School
University of Nottingham
Nottingham, UK

ISBN 978-3-319-87243-8   ISBN 978-3-319-62155-5   (eBook)
DOI 10.1007/978-3-319-62155-5

Printed on acid-free paper

This Springer imprint is published by Springer Nature
The registered company is Springer International Publishing AG
The registered company address is: Gewerbestrasse 11, 6330 Cham, Switzerland

Preface

This book is the third of a three-volume series on the management of the three 'blue light' emergency services (Police, Ambulance and Fire and Rescue Services) published by Springer. There has been increasing contemporary research interest in the leadership and management of the emergency services as the context and challenges of the twenty-first century rapidly change and policy and practice adapt in response. We believe that it appears at a particularly appropriate time in which to take stock, immediately after the European referendum in the UK and as the government legislate to involve directly elected police and crime commissioners in the governance and management of the Fire and Rescue Services in England and Wales.

Historically, and paradoxically, the management of Fire and Rescue Services has been well served by the professional press but has not been well reflected in academic literature. We believe this situation is changing, as interest and demand grow for research on these essential services that are operational in some form in nearly all countries and have existed throughout the world for hundreds of years.

The book is divided into three parts. Chapters 2, 3, 4 and 5 provide a chronological overview of the development of the service in the UK since the New Labour government came to power in 1997 up until the election of a Conservative government in 2015. New Labour adopted a mantra of 'modernisation' for the public services, while the subsequent coalition government adopted 'localism' as its rallying cry. The second part consists of a series of chapters on key managerial issues or themes. These are contextualised by the narrative in the first part but are now explored in more detail. Some, if not all, of these chapters have general resonances across emergency services but are particularly relevant to the Fire and Rescue Services. The third and final part of the book provides some wider perspectives before we take a more general look to the future in the final chapter.

We hope that the book will be of interest to those readers who want a general introduction to the history and management of the Fire and Rescue Services as well as for those who wish to use its contents to explore particular managerial issues either within emergency services or in wider public management. It has

been written so that it can be read in one go or to be read to gain an understanding
of a particular time, subject or issue. Finally, we hope that it will complement and
stimulate interest in the other two titles in the current series.

Nottingham, UK   Peter Murphy
                                                                Kirsten Greenhalgh

Acknowledgements

Like all editors, we owe a huge debt of gratitude to our authors. This book has been for a long time in gestation but not because of any of our contributors – other than ourselves. Academics with knowledge and expertise in the Fire and Rescue Services are, unfortunately, a relatively small band with multiple demands on their time. Our authors have been universally generous and unfailingly patient, and we would formally like to acknowledge and thank them for their contributions.

Secondly, we would like to thank Professor Paresh Wankhade and our publisher Springer, in particular Janice Stern and Christina Tuballes, who have all been both understanding and supportive, and the book could not have reached this stage without them.

We would also like to acknowledge the continuous support, patience and understanding of our respective families (Steph and Rob; Rob, Dan and Josh) who now have a mutual admiration for each other, if not for us!

The authors and publishers would like to thank the following who have kindly given permission to reproduce copyright material:

The *Journal of Finance and Management in Public Services* for use of material in Chap. 4

The *International Fire Service Journal of Leadership and Management*, which published an earlier version of Chap. 8

Every effort has been made to contact all copyright holders, but if any have been inadvertently omitted, we would like to apologise.

Contents

Contributors

Rhys Andrews Cardiff Business School, Cardiff University, Cardiff, UK

Rachel Ashworth Cardiff Business School, Cardiff University, Cardiff, UK

Julian Clarke Edgehill Business School, Edgehill University, Lancashire, UK

Heike Doering Cardiff Business School, Cardiff University, Cardiff, UK

James Downe Cardiff Business School, Cardiff University, Cardiff, UK

Anne Eyre Trauma Training Ltd, Warwickshire, UK

Catherine Farrell Department of Social Sciences, University of South Wales, Pontypridd, UK

Laurence Ferry Durham University Business School, Durham University, Durham, UK

Kirsten Greenhalgh Nottingham University Business School, University of Nottingham, Nottingham, UK

Eddie Kane Institute of Mental Health, University of Nottingham, Nottingham, UK

Steve Martin Cardiff Business School, Cardiff University, Cardiff, UK

Peter Murphy Nottingham Business School, Nottingham Trent University, Nottingham, UK

Anita Pickerden Worcester Business School, University of Worcester, Worcester, UK

Stefan Svensson Division of Fire Safety Engineering, Lund University, Lund, Sweden

Lynda Taylor Nottingham University Business School, University of Nottingham, Nottingham, UK

About the Editors

Peter Murphy is the Professor of the Public Policy and Management at Nottingham Business School. He teaches and supervises at undergraduate, postgraduate, and executive levels. Peter is the Vice Chair (Research) of the Public Administration Committee of the Joint Universities Council, and a member of the Advisory Board of the Centre for Public Scrutiny. His current research focuses on public policy, and in particular the public assurance, performance management, governance, scrutiny, and value-for-money arrangements of locally delivered public services.

Between 2000 and 2009 Peter was a Senior Civil Servant in Whitehall, where he held a series of posts in the Department of the Environment Transport and Regions; the Department of Transport Local Government and Regions; the Office of the Deputy Prime Minister; and the Department of Communities and Local Government. For 5 years he was also a Director of the Government Office for the East Midlands. Prior to joining the Civil Service, Peter was the Chief Executive at Melton Borough Council in Leicestershire. He has been responsible for emergency planning and responding to emergencies at local, regional, and national levels.

Kirsten Greenhalgh is an Associate Professor at Nottingham University Business School. She is currently the Deputy Director of undergraduate programmes and Course Director of the BSc Finance, Accounting and Management. Her current research focuses on strategic management accounting and public and emergency services. Her specific interests are in performance measurement and management and the integrated delivery of services and financial management regimes across the public sector.

Prior to joining the Nottingham University Business School she was a senior lecturer at Nottingham Trent University for 14 years. Her professional background is in management accounting and she is a member of the Chartered Institute of Management Accounting for who she sits on the Adjudications Working Party. She has held a number of management accounting posts in both the National Health Service and Local Government prior to engaging in academia.

Peter and Kirsten have both been on the Editorial team of the *International Journal of Emergency Services*.

Chapter 1
Introduction

Peter Murphy and Kirsten Greenhalgh

This book is the third of a series on the management of the three 'blue light' emergency services, that is, Police Ambulance and Fire and Rescue Services. Following this brief introduction, it explores some of the contemporary issues in the leadership and management of the fire service in the context of the late twentieth and early twenty-first century. This has been a period of major changes in the management of the emergency services in general and the Fire and Rescue Service in particular. As we write, it also appears to be giving way to a new era for Fire and Rescue Services, at least in England. The leadership of local services is effectively being transferred through the 2016 Crime and Policing Bill to directly elected mayors or to police and crime commissioners. This seems therefore like an appropriate time to take stock of the last 20 years.

The book is not, however, meant to be a management handbook for fire professionals. It does not cover many of the things that are integral to the fire service and to firefighters. For example, it does not deal with fire or chemical engineering or with the science and manufacturing of resistant materials. It does not stray into the psychological challenges of stress, anxiety and trauma, which are unfortunately inevitable consequences of some of the situations firefighters often find themselves in. Similarly, it does not deal with equipment, machinery and appliances or with operating standards and procedures. All of these, we believe, are already much better catered for by other authors and publications.

Despite an extensive and voluminous professional press, Fire and Rescue Services are not well served by the academic literature relating to public management or public leadership. The fragmentary nature of emergency services research together with the strong theory-practice divide was one of the reasons for the recent

P. Murphy (✉)
Nottingham Business School, Nottingham Trent University, Nottingham, UK
e-mail: Peter.Murphy@ntu.ac.uk

K. Greenhalgh
Nottingham University Business School, University of Nottingham, Nottingham, UK

© Springer International Publishing AG 2018
P. Murphy, K. Greenhalgh (eds.), *Fire and Rescue Services*,
DOI 10.1007/978-3-319-62155-5_1

1

establishment of the *International Journal of Emergency Services*. Fire services have a rich history that has attracted industrial relations scholars but less interest from public management scholars.

This is very surprising to the editors. Two of the things that make studying the Fire and Rescue Services so attractive are the services' long attachment and strong adherence to evidence-based policy making, and the dichotomous challenge of managing the service when it is in 'response' mode, and managing it when it is promoting public protection, prevention and fire safety within homes, workplaces and communities. Although the culture of the service has not always recognised this dual responsibility or the equal importance of these complementary roles, they do call for quite different combinations of leadership and managerial skills.

Good leaders and competent managers need both sets of these skills. This is increasingly being recognised across all of the emergency services. The ever-increasing complexity of the incidents and emergencies that the three services are being called to respond to also adds to the imperative for greater interoperability and closer collaboration between the emergency services and their personnel.

The adherence to evidence-based policy making and robust justifications for changes in standards and practice is one of the characteristics that could usefully be adopted in other public services. There is no doubt that if things go wrong, the ultimate possibility of a coroners' court or a judicial review interested in facts, evidence and apportioning responsibility has been a strong historical influence on the fire service. However, restating the need for evidence-based policy is a comforting factor for public servants like ourselves when the government is proposing to bring more politics into the leadership of the service.

Our final chapter looks a bit more into this particular crystal ball, ably abetted and prepared by Professor Kane's account of part of its antecedents in Chap. 6.

The remaining parts of this chapter will describe the contents of the chapters leading up to our look to the future, after which we will briefly set out the origins and antecedents of the British Fire Service and its development up to the end of the twentieth century.

The next three chapters trace the chronological story of the fire services. In Chap. 2, we look at one of the most turbulent periods in the history of local government in England and fire services in particular. This saw 'an unprecedented attempt by central government to transform the politics and performance of English local government' with the result being 'a decade of unprecedented change, which had profound implications for the governance of local communities and management of local services' (Downe and Martin 2007).

Chapter 2 recounts one of the most interesting but surprisingly confusing stories of the labour governments' period from 1997 to 2005. The governments' initial 'modernisation' agenda was generally welcomed by other public services. However, much-needed and acknowledged changes in the fire services were slower to materialise and firmly resisted. As we will see from Chap. 3, by the time labour left office in 2010, the fire service had become positively and proactively engaged in the service-improvement agenda and was focussing on prevention, protection and collaborative working across public services. Chapter 2 focusses on the complex and fascinating earlier period of 1997–2005, which was dominated by the national strike and problems with industrial relations.

In Chap. 3, we examine the experience and performance of the newly renamed 'Fire and Rescue' Services in the period 2005–2010. This period extended across the final 'New Labour' administration of Tony Blair and the period from 2007 when Gordon Brown was the prime minister. Unlike the previous turbulent years, this was a period of consolidation and relative stability. Issues of performance management, service improvement, collaboration, and prevention and protection increasingly came to be the services priority.

In Chap. 4, Murphy and Ferry examine the experience in the period 2010–2015. Conservatives and the Liberal Democrats led the first coalition government of modern times. Radical change for public services was back on the agenda and the Fire and Rescue Service was no exception. National economic policy resulted in ever-longer restrictions on public expenditure and an era of austerity, originally envisaged as being for 2 years, in reality dominated public service delivery throughout the 5-year administration (and beyond). The experience of the service under the coalition government is the focus of more detailed analysis and discussion in the following chapters. This chapter provides an overview of the years 2010–2015, to allow these discussions to be appreciated within the overall management development and experiences of the service during the coalition years.

By the time of the election in May 2010, performance management and service improvement were still a high priority, but the 2008 recession and significant reductions in public expenditure were dominating local and national politics. As James Downe and his colleagues recall in Chap. 5, the incoming government promoted 'localism' and a 'sector-led approach' to performance improvement in the Fire and Rescue Services. It was also looking to make swinging reductions to the finances of all local services and virtually demolishing the 'improvement' infrastructure developed by the previous administrations.

The abolition of the Audit Commission, which conducted the Best Value and Comprehensive Assessment regimes, allowed, or in reality required, the sector to take more responsibility for their own regulation and performance. This chapter evaluates the effectiveness of the 'operational assessment and fire peer challenge' which became the key element of the sector's new approach to performance improvement.

Another area that the coalition government was not satisfied with was the nature and extent of collaboration or interoperability between the emergency services. Chapter 6 outlines the findings of research by Parry, Kane, Martin and Bandyopadhyay (2015) commissioned by the government. This report examined the extant landscape of collaboration and suggested ideas and options for future service redesign and rationalisation. In this chapter, one of the authors of the report, Eddie Kane, outlines their key findings, considers the impact of the new service design proposals and examines some of the issues and options for realising its benefits.

After a brief introduction and a look at a range of conceptual considerations that provide a context for discussing FRSs' accountability, Julian Clarke, in Chap. 7, raises a question common to all democratic politics, namely what kind of accountability are we promoting? Accountability to local populations emerged as a fully formed but vaguely defined duty for FRS in the latest 2012 National Framework. Clarke tracks back to find the source of this duty and looks at the emergence of accountability as a central feature of local governance. But one of the central problems of prioritising public services, whether in an era of austerity or of plenty, is the divide between expert allocation of scarce resources and a range of localised 'community' interests which may or may not be consistent with each other. The second part of the chapter discusses this issue and alternative accountability mechanisms.

Anne Eyre, in Chap. 8, explores the phenomenon of heroism in the context of behavioural responses to disaster. Heros and heroism are probably more associated with firefighters and firefighting than any other profession. Drawing on social, scientific, media and health and safety, Anne reflects on the impact and consequences of being labelled a 'hero'. She then considers the implications of heroism for the emergency services arising from recent cultural and legal developments within the UK. The chapter calls for a more informed understanding and debate about the meaning and implications of heroism, particularly in emergencies and disasters.

In Chap. 9, the first of three to look, in more detail, at HRM issues, Anita Pickerden addresses the issue of increasing numbers of older firefighters which, for the purposes of this chapter, covers those who may retire at an age beyond the traditional retirement age of 50. In the past, the firefighters' pension arrangements made it uneconomical for firefighters to continue working for more than 30 years. The abolition of the Default Retirement Age in 2011 and gender equalisation have paved the way for the proposed pension changes. The proposed changes were strongly opposed by the Fire Brigades Union, who feared that older firefighters would not be physically fit enough to perform their duties, thereby putting their service and the safety of the public at risk. Politics aside, it is clear that the Fire and Rescue Services will be faced with an ageing workforce over the next few years, and many of those employees will be firefighters. Anita poses the question!

As earlier chapters demonstrate, the UK government has made a concerted effort to modernise the way in which fire services are managed and staffed. In Chap. 10, Rhys Andrews and Rachel Ashworth consider the introduction of new duties around fire prevention, reformed pay structures, the integrated development programme for fire service personnel and a renewed emphasis on positive working conditions. One important element of this agenda for change has been an emphasis on increased representation of women and minority ethnic people among fire service employees. Reform of human resource management (HRM) practices was regarded as a key policy tool in the drive to make fire brigades more representative of, and responsive to, the communities that they serve. HRM reform was largely undertaken through the introduction of the Integrated Personal Development System (IPDS), which sought to reduce the ambiguity around the roles of all fire service staff at every stage in their professional development, from entry to retirement. Crucially, the IPDS that was introduced to ensure career progression was linked to ability rather than rank and hierarchical position.

In our second chapter on contemporary HRM issues (Chap. 11), Julian Clarke looks at equality, diversity and multiculturalism in Fire and Rescue Services and how the service has responded to serving the increasingly diverse nature of local communities. He examines the way in which the FRSs have attempted to develop and manage improved relationships with minority groups following the publication of the Macpherson report into the death of Stephen Lawrence in 1993 (Home Office 1999) and the inclusion of the Human Rights Act into UK legislation. In an era of declining resources, instant mass communication, 24 h news and the burgeoning influence of social media, FRSs have been required to adapt the way they relate to their public and local communities. He illustrates his exploration with national and local case studies drawn from various attempts by FRSs to both engage more closely and to broaden the range of services and activities they offer to the public.

In Chap. 12, Catherine Farrell focusses on the under-researched area of governance in the Fire and Rescue Service. The fire and rescue authority (FRA) is currently the governing body or board for the vast majority of Fire and Rescue Services (FRSs), and their role in terms of its governance has largely been neglected by academics. Very little is known about how governance operates in practice within fire and rescue authorities. With the advent of police and crime commissioners, this may well change, and this chapter seeks to bring the topic area under much-needed greater scrutiny.

The final two chapters in the main part of this book are concerned with the organisation of Fire and Rescue Services in places other than in England. Chapter 13, by Lynda Taylor, Peter Murphy and Kirsten Greenhalgh explores how and why the Scottish Fire and Rescue Services have evolved since the Scottish Parliament was established in 1999 and more specifically since 2010, when the purpose, legislation, structure, objectives and performance of fire services all started to diverge from their English equivalents. Although Scotland is still partially regulated by UK-wide legislation, such as the Civil Contingencies Act (2004), the country enacts its own legislation on the delivery of most public services, including fire and rescue services. Scotland was not subject to the Fire and Rescue Service Act of 2004 but had its own (very similar) Fire and Rescue Services Act of 2005. The more recent Police and Fire Reform Act (2012) culminated in the establishment of both a single national Fire and Rescue Service for Scotland and new Fire and Rescue Framework in 2013 and an updated one in 2016 following the service restructuring.

The Fire and Rescue Service in Sweden is primarily regulated by the Civil Protection Act and the Civil Protection Regulation which is primarily concerned with protection of the public against accidents. As Stefan Svensson explains in Chap. 14, the legislation is designed to provide reasonable protection against accidents to people, property and the environment throughout the country, taking into account local conditions. The national government cannot make any decisions about the level of protection locally. The legislation is a framework, which includes basic values and principles and to a lesser extent some detail about what should be done and how this should be accomplished but these arrangements have to be agreed with the local self-governing system.

In our final chapter, we describe and discuss some of the changes and proposals that have emerged in 2016 and look briefly to the future. The change of prime minister occasioned by the result of the referendum on membership of the EU has accelerated the passage of the 2016 Crime and Policing Bill with its proposals for police and crime commissioners to take direct responsibility for Fire and Rescue Services. The legislation also proposes to establish an independent inspectorate, new national standards and a new and more transparent accountability framework. However, the details and the implementation of these proposals will be a subject for future authors. The end of 2016 provides us an appropriate place to close our narrative.

A (very) Brief History of the Development of Fire Services from the Eighteenth Century to the End of the Twentieth

Although most of the individual fire services and brigades have their own local biographers, the academic historical literature of the British Fire Services is largely undeveloped (Ewen 2010). The industrial revolution and the commercial needs of the late eighteen and early nineteenth centuries led to the municipalisation and creation of a paid fire service in the UK. As Shane Ewen explains in his history of the British Fire Service, the 'Great Fire' of Edinburgh in 1824 and the appointment of James Braidwood as Master of Fire Engines led to significant structural and functional improvements in the city's firefighting capacity and ultimately to the creation of the first truly organised paid fire service.

Braidwood also instigated the four principals of effective firefighting, which he later disseminated through the publication of his first manual 'On the Construction of Fire Engines and Apparatus, the Training of Firemen and the Method of proceeding in Cases of Fire' in 1830 (Braidwood 1830). These four principles, which became known as the 'Edinburgh model', would generally be recognisable by the service today. The principles were

- Centralised control of the service
- Standardised appliances and equipment
- Identification of the source of a fire and tackling it at source if possible
- Deployment of a disciplined, well-trained and regularly drilled body of firemen

Following a series of uncontrollable and devastating fires across London in the early 1820s and the publication of his manual, Braidwood himself was appointed as the first superintendent of the London Fire Engine Establishment in 1832 just in time to watch the House of Parliament burn down in 1834. Both had a critical impact and accelerated the creation, development and municipalisation of organised fire services in all the major industrial cities and towns in the UK.

In the decades that followed, the idea of the fireman as a working-class hero doing his dangerous duties in difficult circumstances became synonymous with the late Victorian and Edwardian periods, in both the UK and further afield.

The latter part of this period also saw the rise of the Chief Fire Officer and his personal influence, the continued professionalisation of the service, the networking of services across the country and the collective organisation of both senior officers and other staff. In effect, the 'transformation of the fire service from a disparate collection of fire brigades into a cohesive profession at the turn of the twentieth century' (Ewen 2010, p.9).

The two final phases of formative development unsurprisingly came around the periods of the Great War and its aftermath, and immediately before and during the early part of the Second World War.

During the first period, the strong public service ethos of the service was driven by the chief fire officers themselves and strongly promoted from within by all ranks of the service. Similarly, historical associations and the fact that the service had to negotiate with the Home Office also encouraged the influence and the adoption of a 'service' model with many similarities to the model developing in the police. By the outbreak of the Second World War, fire services had become 'an integrated part of the fabric of local government'.

The devastation of the London Blitz led to the temporary creation of a National Fire Service between 1941 and 1947. There was a steep learning curve for the new service, as wartime firefighting required much more strategic deployment of resources, inter-brigade co-operation and more sophisticated risk assessment. Fire services in the major cities could not deal with every single blaze, and they were continually liable to bombs falling on them in the course of their duty.

The wartime experience also led to the creation of the pre-2004 traditional fire services. These have their origin in the 1947 Fire Service Act, which made provisions to 'transfer fire-fighting functions from the National Fire Service, established during the war years, to fire brigades maintained by the councils of counties' (Fire Services Act 1947, p.1). The war also meant that women entered the service for the first time albeit as wartime auxiliaries.

Throughout these phases of its development, leadership and management of the service was dominated by the traditional model of public administration that was to prevail through much of the early and middle parts of the twentieth century. The traditional model of public administration emerged in the UK in the middle of the nineteenth century and was greatly influenced by the writings of Woodrow Wilson in the USA and by Max Weber who set out the theory of bureaucracy in Europe. To these were added the scientific management principles of F.W. Taylor and the fundamental principles of public service policy, principle-agent theory and public service delivery. These were established and universally applied to Fire and Rescue as well as to the remainder of the public services at both national and local levels.

In 1974, there was a comprehensive reorganisation of local government in England and Wales (outside of London). A uniform two-tier structure was introduced, abolishing the previous single-tier arrangements in counties and county boroughs. Several of the historic counties disappeared, new counties were created, and there were widespread boundary changes. Both the territorial police services[1] and fire services changed their boundaries to coincide with the new administrative areas and six of the new counties – Greater Manchester, Merseyside, Tyne & Wear, West Midlands and West and South Yorkshire – became metropolitan counties. Although the geography may have changed the legislative underpinning, the operational practices and the culture of the services remained largely intact.

Even more surprisingly, this remained the case throughout most of the years of the Thatcher and Major governments from 1979 to 1997. While local government and its key major services endured successive waves of significant changes to legislation, objectives, financing, governance and operating environments, not least because of the introduction of Compulsory Competitive Tendering across both blue and white-collar services, Fire and Rescue Services appeared relatively immune to most of these influences. Throughout the period from the Second World War through to 2001, responsibility for fire services rested with the Home Office. Frank Burchill's review into the machinery for determining the conditions of service in the sector quoted in Chap. 2 was not an exaggeration.

> There has been an almost total lack of real political engagement in the fire services since the last firefighter's strike in 1977. The 1947 Act is hopelessly outdated. Local Authority employers of fire brigades have, in general, shown a lack of leadership and purpose especially when acting together to negotiate pay and conditions. The Fire Brigades Union, while professing its enthusiasm for change, has shown no real commitment to making it happen from the centre and in many parts of the has mounted sustained and energetic opposition to change. The senior management of the Fire Service has shown a collective lack of leadership. (Burchill 2000, p.3)

Notes

1. In addition to the 42 territorial police forces (often known as constabularies), there are a number of specialist forces, such as the British Transport Police, the harbour and ports police, the National Crime Agency and the Serious Fraud Office; they did not change their boundaries at this time.

References

Burchill, F. (2000). *Report of the independent inquiry into the machinery for determining firefighters' conditions of service*. London: HMSO.
Braidwood, J. (1830). *On the construction of fire engines and apparatus, the training of firemen and the method of proceeding in cases of fire*. Edinburgh: Oliver Boyd.
Downe, J., & Martin, S. (2007). Joined up policy in practice? The coherence and impacts of the local government modernisation agenda. *Local Government Studies, 32*(4), 465–488.
Ewen, S. (2010). *Fighting fires: Creating the British fire service, 1800–1978*. London: Palgrave Macmillan.
Parry, J., Kane, E., Martin, D., & Bandyopadhyay, S. (2015). *Research into emergency services collaboration 2015 emergency service working group research report*. London: TSO.

Chapter 2
The Gathering Storm: Modernisation, Local Alignment and Collaboration. Fire and Rescue Services Under the Early New Labour Administrations from 1997 to 2005

Peter Murphy and Kirsten Greenhalgh

Introduction

This chapter looks at one of the most turbulent periods in the history of the local government and fire services in particular in England. It was a period that saw 'an unprecedented attempt by UK central government to transform the politics and performance of English local government' with the result being 'a decade of unprecedented change, which had profound implications for the governance of local communities and management of local services' (Downe and Martin 2007). How this agenda played out in the fire services is one of the most interesting but surprisingly confusing stories of the period from 1997 to 2005. Modernisation during this period was generally regarded more positively in other public services, such as local government and the NHS, and much needed changes in the fire service were slower to materialise. As we will see from the next chapter, by the time New Labour left office in 2010, the fire service was much more positively engaged in a public service improvement agenda focussing on prevention, protection and collaborative working across public services. This chapter focusses on the complex and fascinating earlier period of 1997–2005.

When Tony Blair's New Labour government took office after the landslide election of 1997, responsibility for the fire and rescue services in England, Scotland and Wales was part of the Home Office's portfolio. The service in Northern Ireland, which had been a single Fire and Rescue Service since the Belfast Fire Brigade and the Northern Ireland Fire Authority amalgamated in 1973, was the responsibility of the Northern Ireland Office. Northern Ireland was still under 'direct rule' from Westminster and the Good Friday Agreement of 1998 had yet to be signed.

P. Murphy (✉)
Nottingham Business School, Nottingham Trent University, Nottingham, UK
e-mail: Peter.Murphy@ntu.ac.uk

K. Greenhalgh
Nottingham University Business School, University of Nottingham, Nottingham, UK

© Springer International Publishing AG 2018   9
P. Murphy, K. Greenhalgh (eds.), *Fire and Rescue Services*,
DOI 10.1007/978-3-319-62155-5_2

The relationship between the Home Office and the (then) Fire and Rescue Brigades could be characterised as one of 'benign neglect'[1] (Murphy and Greenhalgh 2013; Raynsford 2016). The Home Office agenda and its media coverage was dominated by criminal justice, immigration, the prisons and the security services, all of which enjoyed a higher priority with the government of the time. Successive Home Secretaries and the fire services themselves were content to accept a low (some would say almost subterranean) profile. This is also a reasonable characterisation of the relationships between local fire brigades and the vast majority of local fire authorities as well as the relationship between local fire services collectively with the Local Government Association and its predecessors. Fire and Rescue Services had been allowed to quietly ossify and they were ill prepared for the approaching 'modernisation' storm.

The legislative basis for the service in essence, remained the 1947 Fire Services Act, which transferred the functions of the short-lived, National Fire Service, created as part of the response to the Blitz during the Second World War, back to local authority control. The Fire Services Act 1959, dealt primarily with pensions and staffing, and there was then no additional primary legislation prior to the New Labour administration coming into power in 1997. Various changes to the structure of local government, including the comprehensive reorganisation of 1974, caused barely a ripple in the services as the governance and management of the service elided into the new local authorities.

This primary legislative inactivity was also reflected in a paucity of secondary legislation, policy guidance and performance data and information. The Audit Commission, following its creation in 1983, and prior to 1997, produced only two reports and a management handbook,[2] (Audit Commission 1986, 1995a, b) of fire services, despite the services being part of the annual collection of local authority performance data since its inception in 1993/94[3] (Audit Commission 1995c).

In terms of the response to widespread emergencies, disasters and major incidents, it is sanguine to quote the Civil Contingencies Act. 'Part 2 of the Act updates the 1920 Emergency Powers Act to reflect the developments in the intervening years and the current and future risk profile'. The framework for cooperation and collaboration with the other emergency services was as neglected as the legislative and policy parameters for the service itself.

---

[1] Nick Raynesford was the minister responsible for the Fire Services from 2001 to 2005. Chap. 9 of his book relates specifically to his experiences with the fire service. His opening line states 'This won't take much of your time'. The policy is benign neglect' a quote from Home Office officials handing over responsibility for the service in 2001. Raynesfords' book provides the political and ministerial perspective that complements this chapter.

[2] In 1986, the Audit Commission published *Value for Money in the Fire Service: Some Strategic Issues to be resolved* followed in 1995 by two related reports, *In the Line of Fire: Value for Money in the Fire Service – The National Picture*, and *In the Line of Fire: a Management Handbook on Value for Money in the Fire Service.*

[3] Audit Commission *Local Authority performance Indicators [1993/94]: Volume 3 Police and Fire Services 1995.*

The Themes for This Chapter

This chapter reviews the experience of the fire service under the first two New Labour (1995–2005) administrations. In order to focus the account, it will adopt three themes, although these themes clearly overlapped and were interrelated. The three themes are those included in the chapter title namely

- Modernisation
- Local public service alignment
- Inter-agency partnership and collaboration

Prior to 1997, the service had suffered, as noted above, from a lack of direction from central government. Since 1976, it also suffered long-term under-investment from both central and local government which allowed outdated policies and practices, particularly in terms of its industrial relations, to generate an insular and defensive organisational culture. A series of reports into major disasters and emergencies also meant it was losing its reputation and the confidence of the public. It was about to change, albeit unwillingly.

The period from 1997 to 2005 was a period of turbulence and unprecedented hostile industrial relations. It also saw some of the biggest changes in the service, as it culminated with the enactment and implementation of the 2004 Fire and Rescue Services Act and the 2004 Civil Contingencies Act. This chapter attempts to chronicle these changes, while the following chapter will discuss the period from May 2005 up until the election of the Coalition Government in May 2010. During the period from 2005 to 2010, the service became more reconciled to the government's agenda and significantly improved its performance and its relationship to the government and the public.

The Gathering Storm (1997–2002)

In 1997, prior to the 1999 Greater London Authority Act, the formation of the London Fire and Emergency Planning Authority and the devolution of services to Scotland, and later Wales, there were 50 fire and rescue services in England and Wales and 8 services in Scotland. They were under local authority control (see Table 2.1). The services varied in size from London and Strathclyde to the Isles of

Table 2.1 Types of fire service in the UK

Type of fire service						
England and Wales					Scotland	Northern Ireland
Year	County	Combined	Metropolitan	London		
1997	16	27	6	1	8	1
2005	16	27	6	1	8	1
2016	15	24	6	1	1	1

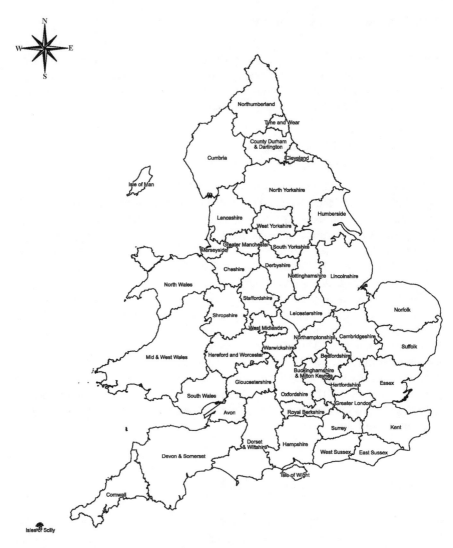

Map 2.1 Fire service in 1997 and 2005 (Source: Ordinance Survey 2016)

Scilly (see Map 2.1) and this number and pattern of local services remained virtually unchanged in the period up to May 2005.

The Northern Ireland Fire and Rescue Service was the responsibility of the Northern Ireland Office and there were a number of smaller specialised and private fire and rescue services. The Ministry of Defence, the Nuclear Authority and the Palace of Westminster all had their own fire services, as did the Airports, the main Ports and some large factories and industrial premises who operated private services.

However, the remainder of this and subsequent chapters are primarily concerned with the local authority controlled services in England and Wales.

The period between 1997 and 2002 saw responsibility for the Fire Service move from the Home Office to the Office of the Deputy Prime Minister (ODPM) via a brief stint in the short-lived Department of Transport, Local Government and the Regions. The responsibility for emergency planning moved from the Home Office to the newly created Cabinet Office Civil Contingencies Secretariat in 2001. It was a period that experienced a complete overhaul of the legislative basis for the service; the second national strike in the services history, and unprecedented upheaval in terms of policy and practice.

However, the Conservatives approach of the Home Office to the Fire Service, which we have characterised as one of 'benign neglect' initially continued. In May 1997, Jack Straw replaced Michael Howard, the outgoing Home Secretary. Howards' tenure had been dominated by his tough approach to crime,[4] and marked by controversies with the judiciary[5] and the prison service.[6] Whether his famous dictum that 'prison works' was true or not is another matter. What is not in doubt was that during his tenure, from 1993 to 1997, prison numbers doubled, from 42,000 to nearly 85,000, and were continuing to increase as a direct result of government changes to sentencing policy. The probation services were struggling to cope and Howard displayed little interest in the fire service.

As Shadow Home Secretary, Jack Straw[7] had an even more authoritarian reputation than Michael Howard. In office, he was soon embroiled in the Steven Lawrence affair and set up the Macpherson Inquiry that was later to find the Metropolitan Police Service was institutionally racist.[8] He also had a new electoral system for the European elections (proportional representation) to introduce and the Human Rights Act to steer onto the statute book. However, one of Straw's first pieces of primary legislation as Home Secretary was to reassert the need for multiple and several organisational responsibility for long-term intractable social problems (which were coined the 'wicked issues'). This Act, and what followed, would radically affect the future scope, form and responsibilities of the fire services.

---

[4] The Conservative Government had sought to hold individual agencies accountable for certain social problems. Howard took the view that tough sentencing and consequential incarceration for longer periods were responsible for the reduction in crime rates during his tenure. His predecessor Kenneth Clarke argued that more effective policing, and better individual, household and car vehicle security all contributed to the reductions. This view was supported by the rising recidivism rate for recently released prisoners which had reached 60% by 1997.

[5] Following his intervention to attempt to increase the minimum sentence of Robert Thompson and Jon Venable for the killing of James Bulger, Lord Donaldson a former master of the Rolls, famously described it as 'institutionalised vengeance by a politician playing to the gallery'.

[6] In 1997, he was accused of interfering in the dismissal of the Director of the Prison Service Derek Lewis.

[7] Concerned about street crime, he had even called for a curfew on children in 1995.

[8] Sir Ian Macpherson Inquiry into the matters arising from the death of Stephen Lawrence.

Collaboration and Alignment of Local Agencies

The 1998 Crime and Disorder Act is more famous for its introduction of sex-offender, antisocial and parental orders, but the conceptual thinking and theoretical underpinning that the Act also re-introduced, were actually more significant and fundamental changes in the approach to the policy and practice of local service delivery.

By 1997 policy makers and academics were much exercised by long term and seemingly intractable social, economic and environmental issues, the 'wicked issues'. These issues were not, apparently, amenable to single agency solution or even mitigation. They required multiple agencies to work together to adopt a focussed, determined and co-ordinated approach in order to have significant impact.

Crime and the rising levels of disorder in civil society were prime examples. The Act re-introduced two fundamental concepts: multiple and several responsibilities for addressing the problem at the local community level, and the need for joined up policy and delivery at local and national levels of government. Henceforth both the Chief Constable and the Chief Executive of the local authority were made personally responsible for producing and maintaining a crime and disorder audit, a reduction strategy and the establishment and leadership of a local partnership of key agencies. Central and local government would co-produce policy and both would be mutually responsible for public service delivery. The 1998 Crime and Disorder Act was the first example of both joined-up policy and delivery under New Labour, as well as multiple and several responsibility between agencies for tackling economic, social or environmental problems seemingly endemic in local communities.

Collaboration and partnership working were not new but the period between 1979 and 1996 had seen a reduction in the number of formal and informal partnerships that local agencies were statutorily obliged to be actively engaged with. Individual agency and personal responsibility were acknowledged to be appropriate for tackling some issues, but the persistence of crime and disorder, the rise in teenage pregnancies, the stubborn resistance of attainment levels in schools to improve or the increasing inequality of health outcomes required a more collective approach. No longer was it a case of investing in prison or probation, health protection or hospitals, prevention rather than cure. It was now a question of joined up policy and practice, and investment in both sets of approaches. This led to the Labour government's early mantra for local service delivery of 'what matters is what works' (Labour Party 1997). Local authorities, the local NHS, the police and fire services were the core of the Local Crime and Disorder Reduction Partnerships, established by the Act, and many more of the local public service delivery partnerships that were to follow.

Similarly, the 1980s and early 1990s had also seen a series of major incidents, emergencies and disasters that had clearly challenged the capacity and capabilities of the local emergency services, and required much more joined-up planning, reaction and response than the emergency services were able to provide. The Bradford and Kings Cross Fires; the Kegworth and Lockerby air crashes; the Hillsborough crush; the Loscoe methane explosions; and the multiple widespread flooding incidents all emphasised the importance of emergency planning and preparedness as well as a co-ordinated inter-agency response from the emergency services. The end of the 'Cold War' in the early 1990s coincided with this rise in peacetime disasters, and emergency planning moved from a concentration on post-nuclear attacks to preparing for a much wider range of man-made and natural disasters. Multiple agency cooperation, co-ordination and collaboration in response to large or widespread disasters was the only realistic way forward. The three blue light services together with the local authorities were the core of the local emergency planning partnerships, which were to become Local Resilience Forums after the Civil Contingencies Act 2004.

Fire Service Modernisation[9]

At the same time as the seemingly endless series of inquests or inquiries reporting on these disasters was casting a critical spotlight onto the response from emergency services, the new government's demand for 'modernisation' of the public services was growing. Local government and the NHS were in the vanguard of modernisation but criminal justice, the police and the fire service would not escape. Modernisation in the fire service was not the same as modernisation in local government or the NHS. However, the nature and form of fire service modernisation was, inevitably, heavily influenced by local authority modernisation, because fire was a local authority service, and the other services then under local authority control were forging ahead with the governments' agenda.

The details, and the development of the fire sectors complex relationship to modernisation, can however only be understood by looking at the service with knowledge of three critical factors:

- The benign neglect of the fire agenda by the Home Office
- The publication of two very critical independent reports into the service
- The co-incidental release of two government documents, which to this day have generated a conspiracy or cock-up debate, that will probably only be resolved by the official release of confidential papers in years to come

It may have been deliberate, or it may have been a co-incidence, but the day that the white paper on local government modernisation was released was also the day that the government sent a letter to the fire services national negotiators, notifying them that the employers were seeking a more flexible negotiating framework at national

---

[9]The following section leans heavily on our article Performance management in Fire and Rescue Services in Public Money and Management 33:3, 225–232.

level (Burchill 2004). This latter proposal was the source of what was to become only the second national strike by the firefighters unions and the first since the 1970s.

The dispute essentially revolved around, not only pay and conditions of service, but the general principle of devolving determination of pay and conditions from national negotiations to local resolutions. For a long time within the fire service this dispute became synonymous with 'modernisation' and eventually resulted in revised national negotiation arrangements. It really started with the letter in July 1998, although a formal strike was not called until November 2002 and was only resolved in July 2003.

In 1999 Jack Straw appointed Professor Frank Burchill, Keele University's first Professor of Industrial Relations, to conduct a review into the machinery for determining the conditions of service. His subsequent report which was published in 2000 stated:

> There has been an almost total lack of real political engagement in the fire services since the last firefighter's strike in 1977. The 1947 Act is hopelessly outdated. Local Authority employers of fire brigades have, in general, shown a lack of leadership and purpose especially when acting together to negotiate pay and conditions. The Fire Brigades Union, while professing its enthusiasm for change, has shown no real commitment to making it happen from the centre and in many parts of the has mounted sustained and energetic opposition to change. The senior management of the Fire Service has shown a collective lack of leadership. (Burchill 2000 p.3)

In July 1998, the government published the Local Government White Paper *Modern local government: in touch with the people* (DETR 1998), which quickly led to the Local Government Act 1999. This act introduced a general duty of Best Value wherein authorities had to 'make arrangements to secure continuous improvement in the way in which its functions are exercised, having regard to a combination of economy, efficiency and effectiveness'. Public service organisations (or at least those designated as Best Value Authorities) had henceforth to seek to achieve best value in the procuring and delivery of services, and to facilitate the achievement of continuous improvement in all of their activities.

In May 2001, responsibility for the fire service transferred from the Home Office to the short-lived Department of Transport, Local Government and Regions and thence to the more powerful ODPM in May 2002. However, the new duty of Best Value resulted in very few significant service reviews within fire services between 2000 and 2002. In September 2002, immediately after the summer recess, the Deputy Prime Minister, John Prescott, announced the 'Bain' review.

The Bain review which reported in December 2002, as Burchill before it, pulled no punches about the need for the service to change:

> We did not realise until we started this review just how much potential for reform exists in the current Fire Service. We were surprised at the extent to which the fire service has fallen behind best practice in the public and private sector. ...The Fire Service needs to be changed from top to bottom and every aspect of its work reformed to bring it into line with best practice at the start of the twenty-first century. (Bain et al. 2002, pii).

Local Government Modernisation

Between 1998 and 2004, the local government modernisation agenda was central to the reform and improvement of locally delivered public services in England and Wales (Andrews et al. 2003; Martin and Bovaird 2005; Downe and Martin 2007; Morphet 2007; Laffin 2008) and fundamentally changed the relationship between central and local government. In 1999 the Department of the Environment, Transport and Regions recruited a Local Government Modernisation Team of ex-local authority Chief Executives and Senior Officers to advise its Director of Local Government, Andrew Whetnall, on the implementation of emerging policy. Whetnall, a career civil servant who had previously been in the Cabinet Office, had been responsible for the 1998 Local Government White Paper and the 1999 and 2000 Local Government Acts. He was keen to ensure effective delivery, or 'how' policies should most effectively be delivered, as well as the traditional civil service concern with 'what' policy should be delivered. After strengthening the team in November 2000, he had the modernisation team work alongside his career civil servants on the various aspects of modernisation, which are shown in the Table 2.2.

Although local government modernisation has generally been portrayed, in academia, as an exercise in introducing new public management theory, focussing primarily upon performance management regimes, it was much more complex and wide ranging than this in both theory and in practice. Whetnall and his team knew that, if it were to be successful, it had to be based on multiple and mutually reinforcing reforms across policy making, scrutiny and delivery of local government services. Table 2.2 was devised within the department in early 2001 to illustrate the various key work streams to the agenda and their role or focus.

At the same time as the main programmes and projects identified in Table 2.2, above, were being initiated, developed and promoted, a rich ecology of supporting

Table 2.2 Modernisation agenda

Local government modernisation agenda	
Agenda	Initiatives
Legal basis and parameters	The power of wellbeing
A strategic vision (derived from the community rather than the LA)	Local strategic partnerships and community leadership
Objectives and priorities (articulated and measureable)	Community strategies
Efficient, effective and economic service delivery	Best Value and collaborative working
Better decision making	New political structures (executive/scrutiny split)
Probity and openness	A new ethical framework and standards board
Innovation and organisational development	New technology and e-government
A sustainable long-term funding regime	Review of local government finance

Table 2.3 Improvement infrastructure

Local government improvement infrastructure	
Area of interest	Project, programme or organisation
Improving the evidence base for local government policy and delivery	Improvement and Development Agency (IDeA) Local authority observatories (web-based, open and capable of interrogation) Knowledge hubs (web-based, open and capable of interrogation) Employers Organisation (EO)
Improving local government as delivery organisations	Improvement and Development Agency (IDeA) The Local Government Leadership Centre Local Government Specialist Consultants Beacon Council Scheme Local Authority Coordinators of Regulatory Services (LACORS) Register of Accredited Political and Officers Peers Employers Organisation (EO)
Improving interagency collaboration	Improvement and Development Agency (IDeA) The Local Government Leadership Centre Beacon Council Scheme 4 ps (Local government partnerships)
Improving local government as community representatives	Improvement and Development Agency (IDeA) The Local Government Leadership Centre The Standards Board The Centre for Public Scrutiny Register of Accredited Political and Officers Peers

organisations and projects were being established. These were later to become known as the improvement infrastructure. Table 2.3, below, is by no means exhaustive but contains examples of both organisations and projects that were established or significantly developed around this time.

Although these new organisations and initiatives were generated around the local government 'modernisation agenda' it was, of course, intended that all of these initiatives would be applied in the fire service. However, in the early days of 1999–2002, the focus was on neighbourhood renewal, Best Value, changes to political structures, the development of delivery partnerships and the performance of the major local government services principally education, social services benefits administration and waste services. In short, fire services were not a priority until Bain revealed the scale of improvement needed. They were keen to keep a low profile and were much more exercised by industrial relations, terms and conditions of services and workforce development.

By 2001, the team in the DTLR had been also working on five new initiatives. Local strategic partnerships, Local Public Service Agreements, the local e-government strategy, the commissioning of comprehensive performance assessments and preparations and piloting for the intervention by central government in 'failing' or significantly underperforming local authorities or their services. All of these, together with the devolution and regional agendas, came together under the auspices of the Office of the Deputy Prime Minister and John Prescott. All of them affected and were applicable to fire services and authorities.

However, as mentioned earlier, the 'distraction' of the Bain review, the subsequent long-running national dispute, together with the strength of the services' organisational culture, and the partial and weak application of the first performance management regime for fire, meant that the impact of the modernisation agenda was much less influential than in the rest of local government.

After accepting every recommendation in the Burchill Report, a new National Joint Council (NJC) for the UK Fire and Rescue Services was established. From 2000 to 2008 Frank Burchill was its chairman, and the NJC played a key part in the settlement of the dispute. The national dispute dominated this period and even after its resolution in July 2003, it was immediately followed by the introduction of the new Integrated Personal Development System (IPDS) for fire service staff and the development of Integrated Risk Management Planning (IRMP) for the organisations. It was these initiatives that tended to dominate the post-dispute 'modernisation' agenda at the personal and organisational levels rather than Best Value the need for continuous improvement, collaboration across local services, joined-up delivery or the new performance management arrangements that local government had by then embraced.

The new pay deal was dependent upon rapid progress toward the government's broader definition of modernisation and in order to trigger the new pay deal, the Audit Commission was asked to verify progress (Andrews 2010). It was therefore asked to carry out two verification reports in March and September 2004 (Audit Commission 2004a, b). The reports were to 'assess progress by fire authorities in England and Wales in implementing the modernisation agenda as set out in the national pay agreement and the subsequent white paper' (Audit Commission 2004a, p.2). This also allowed the government, the Audit Commission and the authorities themselves to make a judgement as to whether the 47 fire services were ready for the rigours of the comprehensive performance assessment (CPA) process.

The first fire service assessments were carried out in 2004–2005, after the annual single and upper tier local authority assessments of 2002–2005 and the District Council Assessments of 2003 (Audit Commission 2009). The methodology used is summarised in Fig. 2.1 below.

The results were not published until after the election in 2005. As with the local authority assessments before them, the services were allocated a single overarching label and five categories of performance were used (poor, weak, fair, good or excellent). The Audit Commission, who carried out the inspections, also provided a 'direction of travel' judgement, to indicate whether they were improving and the extent of their improvement. The direction of travel included four categories: inadequate, adequate, performing well and performing strongly. This latter making sense only when you remember that the statutory requirement for services to operate was on the basis of facilitating continuous improvement. The first results are summarised in Table 2.4 below.

Outside of the service, it was not generally appreciated that the first fire assessments and the methodology did not address the operational parts of the service

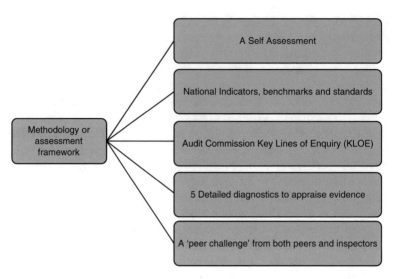

Fig. 2.1 First assessment methodology

(or the performance of the governance arrangements) but only addressed the non-operational parts of fire services (Murphy and Greenhalgh 2013). Neither did it address emergency preparedness, a subject deemed too sensitive by the ODPM at the time. Within the operational parts of the services, the relative ambivalence to the national performance indicators was further compounded by the fact that in 1999 the Home Office had set (and later acknowledged) demonstrably arbitrary targets for some of its key performance indicators. The most notorious was the target for 15% of all operational firefighters to be women by 2009 (ODPM 2004). This would not have been achieved if every new recruit up to and including 2009 were women.

Nevertheless, the ODPM established a means of engaging with those FRAs assessed as poor or weak in order to address the improvement issues identified by the CPA reports published in August 2005:

> Building on experience of establishing lead official roles in local authorities assessed as poor or weak, the ODPM decided to from a small Fire and Rescue Improvement Support Team (FRIST) comprised of external contractors, some of whom had direct experience of providing improvement support in local authorities and others with specialist fire service knowledge... Whilst it drew on earlier guidance and protocols produced for local authorities, specific guidance produced for fire and rescue improvement stressed the aspiration for a voluntary relationship between ODPM and individual FRAs with a focus on the achievement of improvement... Although the possibility of statutory intervention by government is referred to... the prospect was viewed very much as a last resort and a step that would be taken unwillingly. (Coleman 2009, p.1)

As Table 2.3 above shows, by June 2005 there were seven authorities (three combined, three county and one metropolitan) falling into the poor or weak categories: Bedfordshire, Buckinghamshire, the Isle of Wight, Lincolnshire, Northamptonshire, South Yorkshire and Wiltshire. The ODPM established engagement arrangements with all seven authorities.

Table 2.4 The 2005 results

Fire service	Type of authority	Fire CPA score 2005	Fire service	Type of authority	Fire CPA score 2005
Avon	Combined	Fair	Leicester, Leicestershire and Rutland	Combined	Good
Bedfordshire and Luton	Combined	Weak	Lincolnshire	County	Poor
Buckinghamshire and Milton Keynes	Combined	Weak	London	Fire and Emergency	Good
Cambridgeshire and Peterborough	Combined	Good	Merseyside	Metropolitan	Excellent
Cheshire	Combined	Good	Norfolk	County	Good
Cleveland	Combined	Fair	North Yorkshire	Combined	Good
Cornwall	County	Fair	Northamptonshire	County	Weak
County Durham and Darlington	Combined	Fair	Northumberland	County	Fair
Cumbria	County	Fair	Nottinghamshire and City of Nottingham	Combined	Fair
Derbyshire	Combined	Fair	Oxfordshire	County	Good
Devon	Combined	Good	Royal Berkshire	Combined	Good
Dorset	Combined	Good	Shropshire and Wrekin	Combined	Good
East Sussex	Combined	Fair	Somerset	County	Fair
Essex	Combined	Fair	South Yorkshire	Metropolitan	Weak
Gloucestershire	County	Good	Stoke on Trent and Staffordshire	Combined	Good
Greater Manchester	Metropolitan	Good	Suffolk	County	Fair
Hampshire	Combined	Good	Surrey	County	Good
Hereford and Worcester	Combined	Good	Tyne and Wear	Metropolitan	Fair
Hertfordshire	Combined	Fair	Warwickshire	County	Good
Humberside	Combined	Fair	West Midlands	Metropolitan	Good
Isle of Wight	County	Poor	West Sussex	County	Fair
Isles of Scilly	County	Fair	West Yorkshire	Metropolitan	Good
Kent and Medway	Combined	Excellent	Wiltshire and Swindon	Combined	Weak
Lancashire	Combined	Fair			

The Fire and Rescue Services Act 2004 and the Civil Contingencies Act 2004

While relationships between the government, the local authorities and the regulators were undoubtedly improving between 2002 and 2004, relationships between central government and the fire community were significantly deteriorating, following one of the most volatile periods in the services history. 'If 2004 was not the nadir in relationships between the government and the fire community then it was pretty close' (Murphy and Greenhalgh 2014a, p.14).

The white paper that followed the Bain Review *Our Fire and Rescue Services* (ODPM 2003) was as unequivocal as the report that preceded it. The government promised 'a radical overhaul of fire institutions to achieve strategic direction, service improvement and the provision of professional advice' and that it would take powers to determine the number and composition of new negotiating bodies for terms and conditions within the service (ODPM 2003, p.9).

It had specific chapters differentiating national, regional and local responsibilities, institutional reform and the framework for improving performance (Chaps. 4, 5, and 6) and differentiated governance from management when identifying appropriate roles for fire authorities and for fire services (Chap. 7). The Act also changed their name to Fire and Rescue Services.

In our view this was delivered to a:

> *confused, dis-orientated and highly defensive fire community, becoming highly sceptical if not cynical about the intentions of the government of the day. It was also a service that was starting to feel isolated from its key collaborators as its key collaborators, as the other emergency services and wider local service deliverers moved on from arguing about the need for modernisation and began embracing the new era of co-production of policy, and demonstrating improved performance and a willingness to embrace collaborative working.* (Murphy and Greenhalgh 2014a, p.15).

The new Integrated Personal Development System (IPDS) clarified the different roles of whole-time and retained firefighters and permitted direct recruitment into all levels of the service. As Andrews (2010) has noted this linked career progression to ability rather than rank and hierarchical position for the first time.

The Integrated Risk Management Planning (IRMP) process, which is still in operation, required fire authorities rather than the Secretary of State to determine resources levels, both human and capital, in relation to the pattern of risk to the public and the configuration of services (Fitzgerald 2005).

As we state in the article quoted above, the 2004 Act was however the first step in the rebuilding of a mutually respectful working relationship with the New Labour government and a rebuilding of the services historically high levels of trust with the public.

The 2004 Fire and Rescue Services Act and the Civil Contingencies Act 2004 essentially replaced institutions and arrangements, policies and practices that were established by the 1947 Fire Services Act and the 1920 Emergency Powers and 1948 Civil Defence Acts.

Although it was slow and cautious in its implementation, the Fire and Rescue Services Act fundamentally changed the approach to the assessment of risk and subsequent deployment of the service in response to the changing pattern of risks in the community (Murphy et al. 2012; Murphy and Greenhalgh 2014a, b). Prior to 2004, the system based its operations around the risk to buildings and property and used a gravity model to assess its performance in responding to emergency incidents. The 2004 Act and the Integrated Risk Management Planning it introduced, henceforth, required authorities and services to base their risk assessments around the risk to people and communities as well as buildings and places:

> *The new system also reinforced the strong tradition within fire services of policy and decision making based upon a robust and effective evaluation of available data and information, i.e. with strategy and delivery being evidence-led, resting on robust, transparent and quality assured performance data that is systematically investigated and situationally appropriate.* (Murphy and Greenhalgh 2014b, p.37).

The 2004 Act introduced the first National Framework for Fire Services (ODPM 2005), which we describe in the following section. In order to assist services in implementing the new approach, the ODPM provided new databases, tools and techniques designed to help services implement the new IRMP approach. It started developing what became the 2006 FESC Toolkit Review Manual (ODPM 2006) which had been made possible by significant improvements in digital mapping and improvements in IT and computing capacity. The 2004 Act encouraged protection and prevention as well as efficient and effective response. It encouraged greater collaboration and engagement of the services with both emergency service partnerships and wider local delivery partnerships. It also saw a role for the private sector and the third sector, as well as direct delivery by the public sector. Finally, it brought Fire and Rescue Services into the comprehensive performance assessment (CPA) regime.

By 2004–2005, there was a general agreement between central and local government, the local government regulators and inspectorates, led by the Audit Commission, that the introduction of CPA had been a considerable success but that a radical review and updating of the regime was required. Unlike the introduction of Best Value and the first iterations of CPAs (ODPM 2002, 2003), the general principle and desirability of a new version was relatively uncontested.

By 2005, it was generally accepted, albeit grudgingly, that CPA had generated substantial quantitative and qualitative improvements across local government services, as well as significant efficiencies in their running costs (Martin and Bovaird 2005; Audit Commission 2009). Fire and Rescue was about to be brought fully into the agenda.

The Civil Contingencies Act of 2004 was equally radical but also clearly aligned with the governments' new vision for Fire and Rescue Services. Under the Act, fire and rescue services, together with the police and ambulance services', became category 1 responders to all emergencies. The approach was to move from an overriding emphasis on response to a balance with more emphasis on prevention and forward planning, from tackling incidents to creating resilience, from focussing on a risk to property, to the risk to people.

The designated responsible authorities and agencies became jointly and severally responsible for preparing and responding to major incidents and emergencies, and for the recovery of the local communities affected. The previous emergency planning arrangements at national and local authority levels were replaced by more comprehensive 'resilience' arrangements at local regional and national levels. These where to be based on new risk registers and inter-agency planning and response arrangements co-ordinated by national, regional and local resilience boards.

The first decade of the twenty-first century saw a series of major hazards, emergencies and domestic disasters, that unlike the 1980s and 1990s, saw the emergency services at their operational best. The response to these emergencies was to test the new roles, responsibilities and institutions established by the Civil Contingencies Act. They were also going to help restore the services reputation with the government and more importantly with the general public. Cabinet Office Briefing Room A (COBRA) was about to enter the national lexicon.

The First National Framework 2004–2005

In July 2004, immediately before parliament was in pirogue for the summer recess, the ODPM published the first Fire and Rescue National Framework for the year 2004–2005. This attempted the herculean task of bringing all of the various changes and initiatives of the previous years into single document that ran to over 80 pages. It followed a draft published for consultation in December 2003 and Nick Raynesford in his ministerial forward summed up the new approach. Raynesford stressed:

- The shift in emphasis to the prevention of fires was already having significant effects.
- The national framework was a shared strategy that followed a consultation exercise, the response to which had been overwhelmingly positive.
- That the framework, albeit a one-year document, was part of a long-term reform and improvement agenda.
- That the government was committed to achieving long-term reductions in fire deaths and deliberate fires, including real improvement in the most disadvantaged areas, via a new public service agreement.

The framework stresses that this was not a national blueprint. It was to give fire and rescue authorities the flexibility to meet the specific needs of their local communities and, 'a firm foundation on which to build local solutions' (Audit Commission 2005, p.4).

The national framework did not cover Scotland and Northern Ireland as responsibility for fire and rescue services had already been fully devolved. It also anticipated that a forthcoming Fire and Rescue Services Bill would devolve responsibility in Wales to the National Assembly for Wales.

Conclusion

This chapter has sought to show how the fire service changed significantly in terms of its responsibilities and objectives through one of the most turbulent periods of its history. It has sought to chronicle the period from 1997, when Jack Straw inherited a Home Office that had little time or interest in the service up until May 2005, by which time it had become fully engaged with the Labour Governments public reform agenda. In May 2006 the service became the responsibility of the newly formed Department of Communities and Local Government and a succession of Secretaries of State from Ruth Kelly and Hazel Blears to John Denham, although each of these, like Prescott before them, appointed a designated fire minister. If 1997–2005 was a period of turbulent relationships, upheaval and change for the service, 2005–2010 was to represent a period of consolidation and progress.

Raynsford describes this change as:

> *from having been the largely passive custodian of existing standards (no local fire station could be closed without agreement of the Secretary of State) to a new more strategic role, publishing a national framework setting out expectations and giving guidance on how local fire and rescue authorities might respond but leaving individual authorities responsible for their own decisions. An inspection regime, involving the Audit Commission, was put in place to monitor how fire and rescue authorities were responding to the new challenges, using similar methodology to the Comprehensive Performance Assessment while the Fire Service Inspectorate, which had notionally been responsible for this previously was to refocus its work on promoting good practice and supporting the service reform programme.* (2016, p.155)

References

Andrews, R. (2010). The impact of modernisation on fire authority performance: An empirical evaluation. *Policy & Politics, 38*(4), 599–617.

Andrews, R., Boyne, G. A., Law, J., & Walker, R. M. (2003). Myths, measures and modernisation: A comparative analysis of local authority performance in England and Wales. *Local Government Studies, 29*(4), 54–78.

Audit Commission. (1986). *Value for money in the fire service: Some strategic issues to be resolved.* London: Audit Commission.

Audit Commission. (1995a). *In the line of fire: Value for money in the fire service – The National Picture.* London: Audit Commission.

Audit Commission. (1995b). *In the line of fire: A management handbook on value for money in the fire service.* London: Audit Commission.

Audit Commission. (1995c). *Local authority performance indicators 1993/94: Volumes 1–3.* London: Audit Commission.

Audit Commission. (2004a). *Verification of the progress on modernisation: Fire and rescue services in England and Wales.* London: Audit Commission.

Audit Commission. (2004b). *Second verification report on the progress on modernisation: Fire and rescue services in England and Wales.* London: Audit Commission.

Audit Commission. (2005). *Comprehensive performance assessment: Learning from CPA for fire and rescue services in England and Wales.* London: Audit Commission.

Audit Commission. (2009). *Final Score – The impact of the comprehensive performance assessment of local government 2002–08*. London: Audit Commission.

Bain, G., Lyons, M., & Young, M. (2002). *The future of the fire service; reducing risks saving lives: The independent review of the fire service*. Norwich: TSO.

Burchill, F. (2000). *Report of the independent inquiry into the machinery for determining firefighters' conditions of service*. London: HMSO.

Burchill, F. (2004). The UK fire service dispute 2002-2003. *Employee Relations, 26*(4), 404–421.

Coleman, P. (2009). *Fire and rescue improvement: A report prepared for DCLG on the approach and lessons learnt 2005–2009*. (unpublished ODPM archive).

Downe, J., & Martin, S. (2007). Joined up policy in practice? The coherence and impacts of the local government modernisation agenda. *Local Government Studies, 32*(4), 465–488.

Fitzgerald, I. (2005). The death of corporatism? Managing change in the fire service. *Personnel Review, 34*(6), 648–662.

Labour Party. (1997). New labour because Britain deserves better: Britain will be better with new labour. In *The labour party manifesto*. London: The Labour Party.

Laffin, M. (2008). Local government modernisation in England: A critical review of the LGMA evaluation studies. *Local Government Studies, 34*(1), 109–125.

Martin, S., & Bovaird, T. (2005). *Meta-evaluation of the Local Government Modernisation Agenda: Progress report on service improvement in local government*. London: Office of the Deputy Prime Minister HMSO.

Morphet, J. (2007). *Modern local government*. London: Sage.

Murphy, P., & Greenhalgh, K. (2013). Performance management in fire and rescue services. *Public Money & Management, 33*(3), 225–232.

Murphy, P., & Greenhalgh, K. (2014a). Tenth anniversary of the 2004 Acts, FIRE. (pp. 14–16). ISSN 0142-2510.

Murphy, P., & Greenhalgh, K. (2014b). Fire risk assessment – From property to people. *FIRE, 106*, 37–39.

Murphy, P., Greenhalgh, K., & Parkin, C. (2012). Fire and rescue service reconfiguration: A case study in Nottinghamshire. *International Journal of Emergency Services, 1*(1), 86–94.

ODPM. (2002). Comprehensive Performance Assessment – Ministerial Statement, ODPM, Dec 2002. Available at http://www.local-regions.odpm.gov.uk/cpa/statement.htm

ODPM. (2005). *The fire and rescue national framework 2004/05*. London: TSO.

ODPM. (2006). *FSEC toolkit review manual*. London: TSO.

Office of the Deputy Prime Minister (2003). Our fire and rescue service white paper London stationary office.

Raynsford, N. (2016). *Substance not spin: An insider's view of success and failure in government*. Bristol: Policy Press.

Chapter 3
Consolidation and Improvement: Fire and Rescue Under the New Labour Administrations 2005–2010

Peter Murphy and Kirsten Greenhalgh

Introduction

This chapter examines the experience and performance of the Fire and Rescue Services (FRSs) in the period 2005–2010. It included the final New Labour administration of Tony Blair and the period from 2007 when Gordon Brown was the prime minister. Unlike the previous period which was a turbulent period of change when industrial relations and human resource management issues tended to predominate, this was a period of consolidation and relative stability when performance management and service improvement issues increasingly tended to dominate the agenda.

The general election of May 2005 was the third election that the Labour party, under Tony Blair, won. Although its majority in the House of Commons was reduced to 66 seats from the 160 seat majority it had held over the previous 4 years, the outcome was not really in doubt.[1] The liberal democrats saw their share of the popular vote rise and they won more seats than any third party since 1923. Despite losing popularity over the Iraq war, Labour campaigned on the basis of a strong economy, while the conservatives under Michael Howard campaigned on immigration, improving the NHS and reducing crime rates.

The focus on public sector reform and the need to improve public services was a key feature of the campaign that became a central pillar of the new administration. It also featured strongly in the Queen's speech to the opening of parliament:

> My government will build on their programme of reform and accelerate modernisation of the public services to promote opportunity and fairness. My government will bring forward legislation in the key areas of public services delivery: education; health; welfare; and crime. (The Queen's Speech, May 2005).

P. Murphy (✉)
Nottingham Business School, Nottingham Trent University, Nottingham, UK
e-mail: Peter.Murphy@ntu.ac.uk

K. Greenhalgh
Nottingham University Business School, University of Nottingham, Nottingham, UK

© Springer International Publishing AG 2018
P. Murphy, K. Greenhalgh (eds.), *Fire and Rescue Services*,
DOI 10.1007/978-3-319-62155-5_3

The new emphasis on planning, prevention and protection, and the key themes of modernisation, public service delivery alignment and collaborative working across the public sector, established in the previous period (Raynsford 2016), with local authorities in the vanguard, was set to continue and, if anything, become even more influential.

Many of the elements or work steams of the original modernisation agenda, which are shown in Table 2.2 in the previous chapter (p. 17), were built upon and developed between 2005 and 2010. Figure 3.1 attempts to show some (but not all) of the initiatives and their development into the post-2005 period.

The service entered this period under the continuing policy jurisdiction of the ODPM, although in May 2006, departmental responsibilities, including Fire and Rescue, were transferred to the newly created Department of Communities and Local Government under a new Secretary of State, Ruth Kelly. A dedicated fire minister was retained in the new department, but whereas Nick Raynsford had been fire minister for the previous 4 years, the next 5 years, saw five ministers hold the portfolio. Jim Fitzpatrick (2005–2006) a former firefighter was succeeded by Angela Smith (2006–2007), Parmjit Dhanda (2007–2008), Sadiq Khan (2008–2009) and Anne Snelgrove (2009–2010).

The two central 'drivers' of the new government's initial drive to continue to improve local public services individually and collectively, were the second generation of Comprehensive Performance Assessments (CPAs) and the replacement of Local Public Service Agreements (LPSAs) with Local Area Agreements (LAAs) (ODPM 2004a, b; DCLG 2006). Both directly involved the newly renamed Fire and Rescue Services. In addition, 2005 saw the publication of the second National Framework for Fire and rescue services (ODPM 2006), and a new approach to regu-

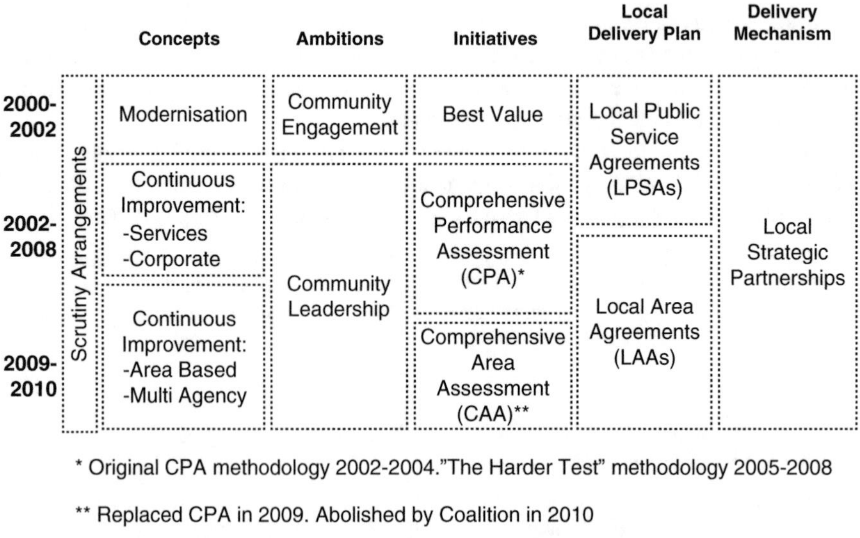
Concepts
Ambitions
Initiatives
Local Delivery Plan
Delivery Mechanism
2000-2002
2002-2008
2009-2010
Scrutiny Arrangements
Modernisation
Community Engagement
Best Value
Local Public Service Agreements (LPSAs)
Continuous Improvement: -Services -Corporate
Comprehensive Performance Assessment (CPA)*
Local Strategic Partnerships
Community Leadership
Continuous Improvement: -Area Based -Multi Agency
Local Area Agreements (LAAs)
Comprehensive Area Assessment (CAA)**
* Original CPA methodology 2002-2004."The Harder Test" methodology 2005-2008
** Replaced CPA in 2009. Abolished by Coalition in 2010

Fig. 3.1 The developing modernisation agenda (Source: Jones 2013)

lation, termed 'strategic regulation' (Audit Commission 2003) and the inspection of public services by all the inspectorates and regulatory bodies for locally delivered public services, summed up in the title of the Office of Public Service Reform (OPSR) report 'Inspecting for Improvement' (OPSR 2003a, b; Davis et al. 2004; Davis and Martin 2008; Downe 2008).

This chapter explores each of these in turn before looking at the final part of the New Labour era under Gordon Brown; when Comprehensive Area Assessments (CAAs) replaced CPA, a second generation of local agreements were agreed and the second National Framework for Fire and Rescue Services 2008–2011 was published. The Brown administration was also the period of the great recession and the onset of austerity and public-sector financial restraints which came to dominate the next period of Conservative-led coalition government between 2010 and 2015.

The 2005–2008 Comprehensive Performance Assessment Regime

Following the 2004 verification reports (Audit Commission 2004a, b) by the end of the second Blair administration, there was a general agreement between the central and local government, the local government regulators and the inspectorates that a radical review and updating of the local government CPA regime was required:

> Unlike the introduction of Best Value and the first iterations of CPA, the general principle and desirability of a new version was relatively uncontested. By 2005 it was generally accepted, albeit grudgingly, that CPA had generated substantial quantitative and qualitative improvements across local government services as well as significant efficiencies in their running costs (Martin and Bovaird 2005). Nevertheless, all parties considered that it could be significantly improved (Martin 2006, Ashworth et al. 2010). There were clearly lessons to be learned from the implementation of the previous regimes, and from the two rounds of Fire Service verifications undertaken by the Audit Commission, as well as from performance management regimes in other sectors such as the police, education and health.
> (Murphy and Greenhalgh 2013, p.227)

The Office of Public Service Reform (OPSR) within the Prime Minister's office had produced its report 'Inspecting for Improvement' as well as the government's new inspection strategy for public services (OPSR 2003a, b; Davis and Martin 2008). The 2005 Comprehensive Spending Review (CSR), and the associated Public Service Agreements for Whitehall spending departments (HMT 2004), had signalled a move to a new set of national objectives for the public sector focused on local outcomes within communities rather than input or output measures for individual public services. They therefore encouraged collaboration across Whitehall departments and sought to re-enforce the connections between public services at the local authority level.

In 2005, 'CPA the harder test' (Audit Commission 2005) was published by the Audit Commission. By this time, as a result of the OPSR reports, the Audit Commission had formally taken on the role of co-ordinating the various inspectorates and regulators that monitored and assessed locally delivered public services (Campbell-Smith 2008). It was also rolling out what it called 'strategic regulation' and envisioning fewer, but more strategic, performance frameworks and inspections across the public services (Audit Commission 2003, 2006).

The new CPA methodology not only looked at how a council was performing as a corporate and service delivery organisation but also as community leaders and collaborative partners to other local services. The new methodology also included a specific service assessment for the Fire and Rescue Services.

CPA for Fire and Rescue Services was to be fully aligned and built on the principles and processes for CPA in local government but it was also intended to address issues specific to fire and rescue authorities. However, because of political sensitivities and the quality and quantity of comparative information available, the first Fire Assessment in 2005 looked only at back-office functions. These were, however, quickly followed in 2006 by assessments of the whole services that included operational services and emergency preparedness as well as back-office services (Audit Commission 2006, 2007).

From 2006, a Fire and Rescue Service Assessment was included in the overall framework for CPA for those 13 councils with sole responsibility for Fire and Rescue Service in their area, and the same methodology was applied to the (then) 32 other combined and metropolitan Fire and Rescue Services and to the London Fire and Rescue Service. Figure 3.2 was the generic diagram used by the Audit Commission to summarise the new CPA framework as a whole, while Fig. 3.3 summarises the Fire and Rescue Service Assessment model.

The 2006 Fire and Rescue CPA was a corporate assessment that attempted to assess performance across both national and local priorities for the service and evaluate the fire authority's response to meeting the needs of the local community. The methodology employed used a self-assessment, completed to an Audit Commission template, a peer challenge (provided by peers, both officers and elected politicians from outside services on the assessments teams) and an external inspection from an Audit Commission team. These assessments were complimented by an evaluation of how economically, efficiently and effectively the services was making use of the resources available to it and an evaluation of whether the service was improving sufficiently rapidly – the latter being called a 'direction of travel' assessment.

All of these judgements were based upon explicit and publically available 'Key Lines of Enquiry'[2] (KLOEs), supported by detailed diagnostic guidance. All elements, together with the scoring and weightings used in the subsequent judgements, were developed in consultation with the government, the local authorities, the fire services and, at least by intention, the public.

The evaluation components and techniques, which are shown in Fig. 3.3, were by 2005 becoming tried and tested parts of the wider regulation and inspection regime within the public sector, although as mentioned above, the initial 2005 assessments were not actually 'comprehensive', as they primarily related to back-office functions.

The early assessments were however, both dependent on a very limited and immature evidential base, as the earlier verification exercises in 2003 and 2004 had revealed. Figure 3.4 gives a four-stage generic typology for the development of evidential

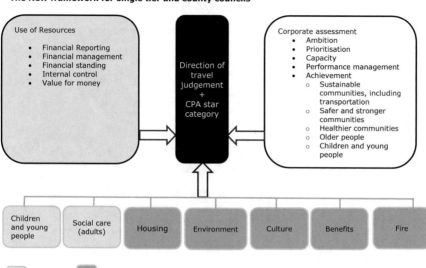

The New framework for single tier and county councils

Fig. 3.2 The 2006 CPA methodology

bases. It was designed for use in performance management regimes and can be applied to individual services, to organisations or to whole sectors. It identifies four 'characteristic' stages, from undeveloped immature information environments (data-poor environments) to robust mature evidence bases (suitable for self-regulation). There are indicative descriptors included for each of the four stages, although in practice, the reality is always likely to be more complicated than the simplistic model implies.

It is, however, clear from this typology that in 2005, despite fire services being part of the Audit Commission's and later the government's successive generations of national performance indicators since they were established in 1995, it still had only a 'data-poor' evidential base from which to operate, benchmark and assess performance and improvement.

In 2005, the 46[3] fire authorities were assessed under CPA and were also required to produce their annual 'Use of Resources' assessments. The results of these are shown in Fig. 3.5 which shows the overall performance and the performance by type of authority. However, the fact is that in 2005, 63% of fire and rescue authorities were only performing 'at or below' minimum standards as shown by the individual authority scores in August 2005 (Audit Commission 2006).

The Audit Commission Assessment concluded that:

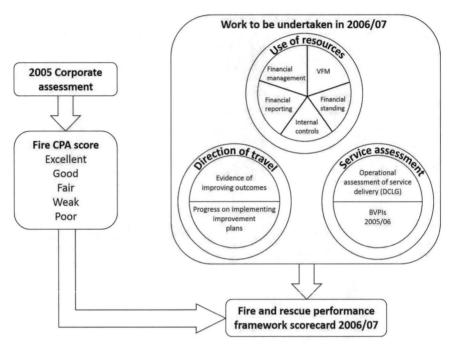

Fig. 3.3 Evaluation components and techniques

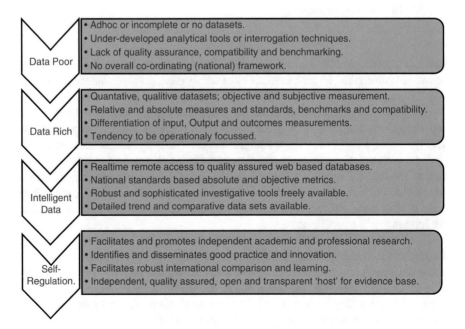

Fig. 3.4 Typology for the development of evidential bases

Authority	Type	Score
Avon	Combined	Fair
Bedfordshire and Luton	Combined	Weak
Buckinghamshire and Milton Keynes	Combined	Weak
Cambridgeshire & Peterborough	Combined	Good
Cheshire	Combined	Good
Cleveland	Combined	Fair
Comwall	County	Fair
County Durham and Darlington	Combined	Fair
Cumbria	County	Fair
Derbyshire	Combined	Fair
Devon	Combined	Good
Dorset	Combined	Good
East Sussex	Combined	Fair
Essex	Combined	Fair
Gloucestershire	County	Good
Greater Manchester	Metropolitan	Good
Hampshire	Combined	Good
Hereford and Worcester	Combined	Good
Hertfordshire	County	Fair
Humberside	Combined	Fair
Isle of Wight	County	Poor
Isles of Scilly	County	Fair
Kent and Medway	Combined	Excellent
Lancashire	Combined	Fair

Authority	Type	Score
Leicester, Leicestershire & Rutland	Combined	Good
Lincolnshire	County	Poor
London	London	Good
Merseyside	Metropolitan	Excellent
Norfolk	County	Good
North Yorkshire	Combined	Good
Northamptonshire	County	Weak
Northumberland	County	Fair
Nottinghamshire & City of Nottingham	Combined	Fair
Oxfordshire	County	Good
Royal Berkshire	Combined	Good
Shropshire and Wrekin	Combined	Good
Somerset	County	Fair
South Yorkshire	Metropolitan	Weak
Stoke on Trent and Staffordshire	Combined	Good
Suffolk	County	Fair
Surrey	County	Good
Tyne and Wear	Metropolitan	Fair
Warwickshire	County	Good
West Midlands	Metropolitan	Good
West Sussex	County	Fair
West Yorkshire	Metropolitan	Good
Wiltshire and Swindon	Combined	Weak

Fig. 3.5   2006 Fire CPA results

Whilst there is a clear appetite for change in fire and rescue authorities the pace varies substantially and improvement has not been achieved to the extent that might be expected..... only a small proportion of fire and rescue authorities are performing across the board at above minimum requirements (Audit Commission 2006, p.2).

In a section on 'next steps for supporting improvement', it adopted the now prevailing collaborative approach to public service improvement. It set out what it anticipated that the government would do to improve the situation, what the commission itself would do, what the improvement organisations would do and what it expected the fire authorities themselves to do. It also gave a foretaste of its proposals for the next round of CPA so that all fire services could better prepare.

The authorities found to be in the lowest 'poor' and 'weak' performance categories became subjected to a central government improvement and intervention regime. This essentially consisted of appointing a 'Lead Official' to act as the chair and co-ordinator of a Government Monitoring Board and provide direct liaison with the government's fire minister. The monitoring board would be responsible for drawing up and implementing an improvement or recovery plan. In so doing, it was to be aided and could call directly upon the resources of the Improvement and Development Agency (IDeA), the Audit Commission and the Local Government Leadership Centre (LGLC) together with assistance from other Fire and Rescue Services and from local authorities. It could also commission services from the private sector, if necessary.

This regime was explicitly built on the 'intervention' model which had been developed for significantly underperforming local authorities and individual local authority services, under the CPA regime since 2002 (ODPM 2003; Jones 2013; Murphy and Jones 2016). The generic model was by this stage robust and well tri-alled and was subsequently applied to other sectors including the NHS.

All of the remaining fire authorities, however, also had available to them capacity and capability, innovation and improvement tools, techniques, programmes and guidance from these same improvement agencies. By the time the CPA results for 2006 were published in late 2007 (Fig. 3.6 below), the majority 37 (80%) of the Fire and Rescue Services were rated as improving 'well' or 'strongly' (the top two categories). In addition, the scores for the annual 'Use of Resources' assessment showed equally impressive improvement.

Although Fire and Rescue Services were initially reluctant and were late to become involved in CPA, it is fair to say that they benefited from the lessons learnt by both the Audit Commission, the government and the local authorities in the early days of CPA (Audit Commission 2006, 2007, 2008a, 2009b). The key stakeholders were therefore able to capture, disseminate, share and apply the lessons learnt, demonstrable good practice and organisational and systemic innovation from their peers. By 2009 when the Audit Commission published its overall assessment of the impact of CPA between 2002 and 2008, few argued with their view that CPA had achieved its objectives of stimulating service improvement and efficiency in Fire and Rescue Services as well as in wider local government (Audit Commission 2008a, 2009a, b; Coleman 2009). In terms of financial improvements, in addition to the annual 2% that HMT assumes will be achieved as a result of technological innovation and other generic improvements, and therefore builds into its annual financial allocations, local government services were making annual cumulative financial savings of between 3% and 4%. Similarly, in terms of service improvement, because of the requirement for continuous improvement and the relative nature of a lot of the national indicators, to attain the same level of performance from 1 year to the next on national indicators, required an actual improvement on average of about 3%.[4] Thus, the improvements in the tables below appear less impressive than the *actualité*.

The quest for continuous improvement was not however over and in 2009 CPA was replaced by a new regime called Comprehensive Area Assessments (CAAs). This was foreshadowed in the 2007 Local Government and Public Involvement in Health Act. In 2008, the government also published the second National Framework for Fire and Rescue Services for the period 2008–2011 which was inter-related with the new CAA regime. However, in order to understand the thinking and philosophy behind these changes, it is necessary to understand the development of a second major driver of public service improvement between 2005 and 2009, namely the Local Area Agreements.

Direction of travel

All fire services have continued to improve in the last year.

Direction of travel category	2006	Change			2007
Improving strongly	2				5
Improving well	30		13		23
Improving adequately	15		5		18
No improvement	0				0
Total fire services	47				46

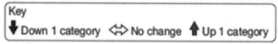

Key
⬇ Down 1 category ⬌ No change ⬆ Up 1 category

Source: Audit Commission

Use of resources scores

Most services (80 per cent) are performing well.

Use of resources category	2006	Change			2007
Performing strongly	3		3		4
Performing well	37		33		37
Adequate performance	7		3		6
Inadequate performance	0				0
Total fire services	47				47

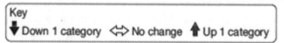

Key
⬇ Down 1 category ⬌ No change ⬆ Up 1 category

Source: Audit Commission

Fig. 3.6 CPA results 2007

Local Area Agreements

Local Area Agreements (LAAs) had been introduced in 2004, as a development of the previous Local Public Service Agreements (LPSAs) between the central and local government. Like their predecessors, they were a mechanism for achieving challenging targets for improved service delivery based on national and local policy priorities. As a reward for achieving agreed performance targets, local authorities and their local partners would receive additional monetary reward and a reduction in central government regulation over particular activities.

LAAs were negotiated with 150 Local Strategic Partnerships (LSPs) rather than with local authorities, although the authorities were expected to lead negotiations on behalf of the partnerships. They were 3-year agreements focusing on revenue rather than capital expenditure and were geographically defined by individual local authority boundaries. From the start, Fire and Rescue Services, who were members of all Local Strategic Partnerships, were also actively engaged in LAAs. In March 2005, the first round of 21 'pathfinder' LAAs were signed off by central government and local area representatives.

In return for achieving mutually agreed 'stretch' targets for improving local delivery of priority services, local area partners would be rewarded through financial incentives and so-called freedoms and flexibilities from central government regulations. Although the objectives, priorities and targets for the first agreements were organised around three 'blocks' of service areas (Community Safety, Children and Young People and Older Peoples Services), this was quickly developed into four slightly more comprehensive blocks that then endured for the life of LAAs. The second round of 66 agreements were signed in March 2006 and the final 62 in March 2007, by which time every large local authority, every Police and Fire Authority and every Primary Care Trust (PCT) from the NHS, together with hundreds of their delivery partners, were working collaboratively across the country to deliver LAAs.

The key issues for individual LAAs arose from the Sustainable Community Strategy[5] for an area, and these were corralled around four baskets of services and activities, universally referred to as 'blocks':

- Safer and Stronger Communities, which were proposals for improving community safety and building more resilient local communities
- Children and Young Peoples Services, which included ambitions such as raising attainment levels in schools or reducing teenage pregnancies in an area
- Healthier Communities and Older Peoples Services which essentially embraced public health, social care and well-being issues
- Economic development, enterprise and innovation in the local economy

Local budgets and efforts were pooled, co-ordinated or rationalised to achieve outcomes agreed on both national and local priorities (see Fig. 3.4). Each of the four blocks had to have agreed outcome targets, sub-outcomes, indicator targets and delivery activities. Three types of funding went into the agreements:

- Mainstream funding from central and local sources which could be aligned against specific LAA outcomes and targets
- Area-specific funding from government departments to local areas which could be pooled in an LAA
- Non-departmental public bodies' (NDPBs) funding which they could choose to align with LAAs (Fig. 3.7)

LAAs led to more effective joining up, co-ordination of local public services and significantly improved outcomes for local communities. They also led to better informed and more economic, efficient and effective government at both the national

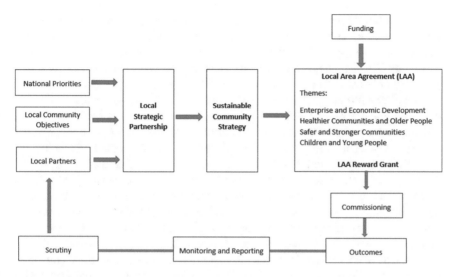

Fig. 3.7 The Local Area Agreement regime

and local levels. Whitehall departments, as well as local delivery agencies, had to strategically align objectives and policies into mutually reinforcing strategies that would lead to improved outcomes for communities.

As the potential success of the three rounds of pilots became clear, the 2006 Local Government White Paper and the Local Government and Public Involvement in Health Act 2007 that followed made LAAs a key performance management and priority setting tool for local areas. Place and place shaping entered the lexicon of national and local government language and a new series of LAAs were a key part of the new ambitions and arrangements.[6]

Local authorities were vested with the duty to lead and enable LSPs in the preparation of new LAAs with much wider partner involvement. The act listed 21 types of organisations with a duty to co-operate and have regard to the targets. It strengthened involvement of the third sector, simplified funding within LAAs and encouraged a move from four blocks (allegedly encouraging a silo service mentality) to four cross-cutting themes. Prevention and protection rather than cure and reaction rose even further up the policy priorities at national and local levels.

Although a new (much-reduced) national indicator set was produced,[7] there was a much greater focus on *local* priorities. A 'dry run' of negotiations was undertaken with 17 areas to generate good practice and ensure a local focus could be maintained. New LAAs had to build a coherent narrative, tell a story and develop the vision of the local 'place'. The local evidential base therefore had to be built and refined[8] to underpin any decisions or targets and justify priorities in negotiations with the central government. Negotiations with central government were conducted through the Government Regional Offices and the whole regime was made open and transparent with a single dedicated publically accessible LAA website, acting as the central repository for all agreements and every target. New Local Area Agreements were successfully agreed for all 150 LSPs as previous agreements reached their termination dates, and a further round was negotiated prior to the 2010 general election and was subsequently implemented over the next 3 years.

In July 2010, immediately after the election, the coalition government's new Secretary of State for Communities and Local Government, Eric Pickles, announced the end of any further LAAs, the abolition of the Audit Commission and the closing of Government Regional Offices. This was followed by the Chancellor George Osborne announcing the (misnamed) 'Bonfire of the QUANGOs' (Quasi Autonomous Non-Governmental Organisations'),[9] which included the dismantling of much of the systemic improvement infrastructure designed to support local authorities, the police, the NHS and Fire and Rescue Services to improve their services to the public.[10]

These abrupt policy changes effectively brought to an end the period of joined up policy and delivery and an era of unprecedented vertical collaboration between central and local government and horizontal collaboration between public and voluntary services within local communities. However, before we examine the coalition government years between 2010 and 2015, we need to look at how these collaborative principles were developed and enshrined in the two National Frameworks for Fire and Rescue Services, which was published in 2005 and 2008 and covered the periods 2005–2008 and 2008–2011. LAAs, crime and disorder partnerships and community safety strategies had encouraged and enabled Fire and Rescue Services to collaborate with local delivery partners, the National Frameworks focused on national and local emergency services and their preparations and responses to local and national incidents.

The National Fire and Rescue Frameworks 2006–2008 and 2008–2011

The second National Framework (DCLG 2006) covered a 2-year period and the third framework (DCLG 2008) covered a 3-year period. The second followed a very similar scope, content and structure to the one adopted for the first framework although it clearly moved on in terms of objectives and targets. The third National Framework was noticeably slimmed down and less prescriptive.

These frameworks attempted to complement and, where possible, integrate with the developing performance management regime for the sector. They were also increasingly the product of co-design between the government and the fire and rescue sector as a whole. Relations between the government and the fire sector and the fire sector and the public both continued to improve, as public satisfaction and regard to the fire sector returned to some of the highest levels of trust and confidence experienced by public services.

With each iteration of the fire service framework, the emphasis on prevention and protection became more pronounced as the performance of the service continually improved. In 2013 the then government Chief Fire and Rescue Advisor, Sir Ken Knight, reflected this in his comment:

It is clear that the cumulative effect of building and furniture regulations, Integrated Risk Management Planning, and the localisation of decision making, and importantly the fire prevention and protection work carried out by fire and rescue authorities has significantly reduced the risk of fire in England. (Knight 2013, p.12)

The second National Framework reflected and complemented the later iterations of the CPA regime, the first generation of LAAs and the final Tony Blair administration. The third National Framework was aligned with the CAA, the second generation of LAAs and the administration of Gordon Brown as the prime minister.

Comprehensive Area Assessment and the New Generation of LAAs

Comprehensive Area Assessments (CAAs) were introduced by the 2007 Local Government and Public Involvement in Health Act, which also heralded a new 3-year Comprehensive Spending Review, a new set of Public Service Agreements for Whitehall delivery departments, a new national indicator set and the second generation of LAAs described above. They were only carried out once and were intended to assess the performance and impact of local public services on local communities in 2008–2009. This impact was to be measured both collectively and individually.

Like the new PSAs, they were intended to be outcome focused and to ensure locally delivered public services were aligned, joined up or integrated wherever possible. They were to be based on collectively agreed local objectives and priorities and to be delivered in the most economic, efficient and effective ways possible. They were also to seek to achieve more sustainable and more equable outcomes for local communities.

CAA was integral to the third National Framework (DCLG 2008) and consisted of an area assessment of the impact or outcomes being achieved collectively by the key public services within a geographical area, complemented by an individual organisational assessment for these key local public service providers. This group included the core members of the Local Strategic Partnership, that is, the local authorities, the Primary Care Trusts (part of whose formal duty was to lead and co-ordinate the local NHS), the local Police Authority and the Fire and Rescue Authority.

For Fire and Rescue Services, it included the first 'operational service assessments' of Fire and Rescue Services (DCLG 2008) and for all parties it included a common 'Use of Resources' Assessment to be carried out by the same external auditors[11] for each of the services in a single area. A new 'Use of Resources' model designed, inter alia, to exclude the shifting of costs from one public service to another was rolled out annually from 2007. It included an assessment of the use and management of all human, financial and physical resources, and it embraced the assessment across short-, medium- and long-term horizons. The 'Use of Resources' assessment had come a long way from the simple assessment of the content and publication of the annual financial accounts in the first CPA in 2001.

In addition to the generic area assessment, specific organisational assessments were developed and carried out on all of the 46 FRS, as well as all local authorities,[12] PCTs,[13] territorial police constabularies,[14] (see Fig. 3.8), with the results published

Strategic alignment across frameworks

Area Assessment
(partnership outcomes)

Organisational Assessment

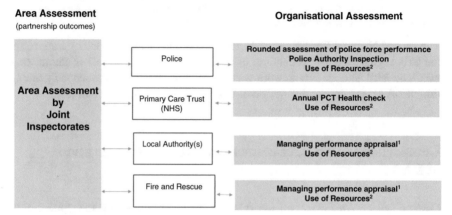

1 Managing performance appraisal (a corporate appraisal of all functions)
2 Use of Resources (which consisted of appraisals of)
   • Managing Finances
   • Governing the Business
   • Managing Resources

Fig. 3.8 CAA methodology (Source: Audit Commission 2008b)

on the Audit Commissions dedicated 'One Place' website which is now only recorded in the web archive of the National Archives.

LAAs became a key part of the area assessment, while an operational assessment, together with the Use of Resources Assessment, became key parts of the FRS organisational assessment.

To facilitate benchmarking, sharing and dissemination of ideas, lessons learnt and good practice, three dedicated, open access, interoperable and real-time websites were established. These were intended to operate as central repositories or 'one-stop shops' for the new Local Area Agreements, for the CAA results and reports (One Place)[15] and by the Local Government Leadership Centre for the 13 innovative pilots that were intended to help facilitate the next stage of development of the improvement agenda for local public services (Total Place).[16]

Conclusion

By 2010, although Fire and Rescue Services had not reached the levels of performance being achieved in local authorities, and clearly had potential for further significant improvement, the annual reports and scores reflected an increasingly engaged and improving sector with an accelerating and positive direction of travel (Audit Commission 2006, 2007, 2008a, 2009a, b). The CAA reports published on the CAA (One Place) website also showed organisational improvement, collaborative improvement and further financial improvement in the year that the CAA system operated.

In early 2010, it was anticipated that the Audit Commission would produce an annual analysis of the results of the CAA process and for the first time have a fully comparable assessment of the use being made of the public resources being expended across local government, health, police and fire services in local communities. The Commission, with the assistance of its regulatory partners, should have been able to report on the quality and quantity of collaboration as well as providing individual service judgements. It should also be able to give the government the public and the public service delivery bodies an idea of the level and speed of improvement of those public services, as well as being able to identify and demonstrate areas of innovation and good practice.

As most readers will know this was not to be, as in the next period, the Audit Commission was abolished, CAA abandoned and no more Local Area Agreements were signed. The emphasis on prevention, protection, service improvement and public service reform in fire as in other public services was about to be succeeded by an emphasis on austerity and reductions in public funding occasioned by a change in political control and macro-economic strategy.

Notes

1. A very late narrowing of the gap in support between the two main parties meant the popular vote was much closer than seats won.
2. Key Lines of Enquiry were originally conceptualised and developed by the former Audit Commission but are now used by most public service inspectorates. They direct the focus of an inspection or assessment onto critical questions or issues. The inspection teams usually publish these in advance and then use a standard set of KLOEs to all of the service delivery bodies.
3. Following the amalgamation of Devon and Somerset, the number of fire services reduced to 46.
4. The calculation of 3% performance improvement on national indicators was a calculation made by analysts on the intervention team when evaluating improvement and recovery strategies. The 3–4% financial savings is a calculation triangulating evidence from the Use of Resources Reports, the schedules of 'Gershon' savings by local authorities and the successive annual 'Invest to Save' programmes. It is little known (except of course by HMT) that the Invest to Save programmes undertaken by local authorities consistently outperformed the programmes of central government departments and non-departmental public bodies (NDPBs).
5. The preparation of a community strategy was a requirement of the Local Government Act 2000. It sets out a long-term vision for an area (which matches the authorities boundaries) and is backed up by action plans to achieve it. Every local authority should prepare a community strategy 'for promoting or improving the economic, social and environmental well-being of their area and contributing to the achievement of sustainable development in the United Kingdom'. The

name generally became the Sustainable Community Strategy during the roll-out of Local Areal Agreements (LAAs) and was formally endorsed in the 2007 Local Government and Public Involvement in Health Act.

6. In addition to LAAs, 'Multi-Area agreements' aimed to encourage cross-boundary partnership working at a geographical scale greater than a single local authority area (either regional or sub-regional). They were not constrained by the 3-year timescale of an LAA nor by including only revenue expenditure. Promoted by DCLG as voluntary agreements between two or more top-tier county councils or metropolitan district councils or unitary local authorities, their partners and the government work collectively to either improve services or address problems best tackled at a larger scale. Often focusing on economic development, the skills agenda and/or transport and access issues, they were forerunners to the current debate on combined authorities. There were 15 signed-off multi-area agreements although there was little involvement by Fire and Rescue services or Authorities.

7. There was a significant reduction in number in national indicators and an improvement in the sophistication of individual indicators throughout this period although the potential scope for further improvements was always clear.

8. The core of the evidential base gradually revolved around the Joint Strategic Needs Assessments, which had been developing since 2004 but found expression in the 2007 Local Government and Public Involvement in Health Act.

9. There were not one 'Quasi Autonomous Non-Governmental Organisations' included on the list at any time, since government by definition did not have control over them. The various iterations of the list consisted of NDPBs and various government advisory groups.

10. Table 3 of Chap. 2 illustrates the nature and scope of this 'improvement' infrastructure. This organisational language was simplified, consolidated and strengthened between 2005 and 2010 but was effectively decimated after 2010.

11. The advantage of having all public services in a single geographical area with the same external auditor was quickly acknowledged as a good idea by government, public service deliverers and the Audit Commission.

12. In areas with the two-tier system of local government, the districts were included in the assessment of the county council.

13. Primary Care Trusts as the formal leaders of the local NHS.

14. Police authorities did not include specialised or national forces.

15. The LAA website no longer exists and a sample from the Audit Commissions 'One Place' website was transferred to the national archives at http://webarchive.nationalarchives.gov.uk/20101008004702/http://oneplace.audit-commission.gov.uk/pages/default.aspx

16. The Total Place website has been dormant for over 5 years but is at http://www.localleadership.gov.uk/totalplace/

References

Ashworth, R., Boyne, G., & Entwistle, T. (Eds.). (2010). *Public service improvement: Theories and evidence.* Oxford: Oxford University Press.

Audit Commission. (2003). *Strategic regulation: Minimising the burden, maximising the impact.* London: Audit Commission.

Audit Commission. (2004a). *Verification of the progress on modernisation: Fire and rescue services in England and Wales.* London: Audit Commission.

Audit Commission. (2004b). *Second verification report on the progress on Modernisation: Fire and rescue services in England and Wales.* London: Audit Commission.

Audit Commission. (2005). *CPA the harder test: framework for 2005.* London: Audit Commission National Report.

Audit Commission. (2006). *Comprehensive performance assessment: Learning from CPA for the fire and rescue service in England 2005.* London: Audit Commission.

Audit Commission. (2007). *Comprehensive performance assessment: Learning from CPA for the fire and rescue service in England 2006.* London: Audit Commission.

Audit Commission. (2008a). *Fire and rescue performance assessment, scores and analysis of performance in fire and rescue authorities 2007.* London: Audit Commission.

Audit Commission. (2008b). *Comprehensive area assessment framework document.* London: Audit National Report.

Audit Commission. (2009a). *Final score – The impact of the comprehensive performance assessment of local government 2002–08.* London: Audit Commission.

Audit Commission. (2009b). *Fire and rescue performance assessment, 2009 – Scores and analysis of fire and rescue authorities performance 2008.* London Audit Commission Community Safety National Report.

Campbell-Smith, D. (2008). *Follow the money – the audit commission, public money and the management of public services 1983–2008.* London: Allen Lane.

Coleman, P. (2009). *Fire and rescue improvement: A report prepared for DCLG on the approach and lessons learnt 2005–2009.* (unpublished ODPM Archive).

Davis, H., & Martin, S. (2008). *Public services inspection in the UK.* London: Jessica Kindersley.

Davis, H., Downe, J., & Martin, S. (2004). *The changing role of audit commission inspections in local government.* York: Joseph Rowntree Foundation.

Department of Communities and Local Government. (2005). *Fire and rescue service National Framework 2005–08.* London: TSO.

Department of Communities and Local Government. (2006). *Strong and prosperous communities: The local government white paper.* Norwich: TSO.

Department of Communities and Local Government. (2008). *Fire and |rescue service National Framework 2008–11.* London: TSO.

Downe, J., (2008). *Inspection of local government services.* Chapter 2 in Davis, H., & Martin, S. Public Services Inspection in the UK London: Jessica Kindersley.

Her Majesty's Treasury. (2004). *Spending review public service agreements 2005–2008.* London: TSO.

Jones, M. (2013). *Corporate recovery and strategic Turnaround in English Local Government.* DBA. Nottingham: Nottingham Trent University.

Martin, S. (2006). *Ed Public service improvement: policies, progress and prospets.* Abingdon: Routledge.

Martin, S., & Bovaird, T. (2005). *Meta-evaluation of the local government modernisation agenda: Progress report on service improvement in local government.* London: Office of The deputy Prime Minister.

Murphy, P., & Greenhalgh, K. (2013). Performance management in fire and rescue services. *Public Money & Management, 33*(3), 225–232.

Murphy, P., & Jones, M. (2016). Building the next model for intervention and turnaround in poorly performing local authorities in England. *Local Government Studies, 42*(5), 698–716.

Office for Public Service Reform. (2003a). *Inspecting for improvement*. London: TSO.

Office of Public Services Reform. (2003b). *The Government's policy on inspection of public services*. London: OPSR.

Office of the Deputy Prime Minister. (2003). *Government engagement with poorly performing councils: Practice guidance for lead officials* (2nd ed.). London: TSO.

Office of the Deputy Prime Minister. (2004a). *The fire and rescue National Framework 2004/05*. London: TSO.

Office of the Deputy Prime Minister. (2004b). *Local area agreements: A prospectus*. London: TSO.

Office of the Deputy Prime Minister. (2006). *The fire and rescue National Framework 2006–08*. London: Office of The Deputy Prime Minister.

Raynsford, N. (2016). *Substance not spin: An insider's view of success and failure in government*. Bristol: Policy Press.

The Queen. (2005). *The Queen's speech to the opening of parliament 2005*. Available at: http://www.publications.parliament.uk/pa/ld200506/ldhansrd/vo050517/text/50517-01.htm.

Chapter 4
Another Turn of the Screw: Fire and Rescue Under the Coalition Government of 2010–2015

Peter Murphy and Laurence Ferry

Introduction

To fully appreciate the coalition governments' approach to Fire and Rescue Services (FRSs), we must contextualise it within public service reform and the wider economic agenda. The global financial crises officially began with the USA entering a recession in December 2007, following a series of housing bubbles around the world and the US subprime mortgage crisis of 2007. Lehman Brothers collapsed on 15 September 2008 and Bear Stearns and Merrill Lynch were already in unavoidable trouble. In the UK, the official start of the recession was the second quarter of 2008, and Gordon Brown announced a bank rescue package of around £500 billion on 8 October 2008. By the time the general election of May 2010 returned a hung parliament and the first modern coalition government between the Conservative and Liberal Democrat parties, local government in general and Fire and Rescue Authorities (FRAs) had been preparing for significant reductions in central government funding for some time.

When annual budgets were being prepared in late 2008, it was the second year of a relatively generous 3-year financial settlement from the government. Nonetheless, the government, the Local Government Association, the Audit Commission and the Society of Local Authority Chief Executives were all strongly advising prudence for local authorities in their short and long-term budgetary planning. As contemporary (Audit Commission 2008, 2009, 2010), and retrospective studies (Lowndes and McCaughie 2013) and international comparisons confirm (Barbera et al. 2014; Steccolini et al. 2014), local authorities reacted positively and rapidly to the challenge

P. Murphy (✉)
Nottingham Business School, Nottingham Trent University, Nottingham, UK
e-mail: Peter.Murphy@ntu.ac.uk

L. Ferry
Durham University Business School, Durham University, Durham, UK

© Springer International Publishing AG 2018   45
P. Murphy, K. Greenhalgh (eds.), *Fire and Rescue Services*,
DOI 10.1007/978-3-319-62155-5_4

of impending austerity as they changed priorities, cut expenditure or built up reserves and, in many cases, did all three, in the period from 2008 to 2010. By 2010, Fire and Rescue Servicess, like their local authority counterparts, had become very robust and resilient organisations[1] in terms of their financial management and service delivery (Walker 2015).

Unfortunately, for public services in June 2010, the new chancellor delivered his emergency budget[2] and was about to embark on an unprecedented series of missed economic and social targets including a target to reduce the (so-called) long-term structural deficit within the life of the parliament. A total of 80% was to come from public expenditure reductions with 20% from the benefits of increased growth. The missed targets not only had an enduring significant impact on public expenditure but also the governments' failure to achieve its targets meant entrenched and persistent austerity became the dominant discourse or narrative of the Coalition administration, and also led to evermore tighter or punitive targets for locally delivered public services:

> This Budget is the first step in transforming the economy and paving the way for sustainable, private sector led growth, balanced across regions and industries........ As a result of the Budget measures the richest will contribute the most to deficit reduction, and the impact on child poverty in 2012-13 is statistically insignificant. (HMT, pp. 3–4)

The LGA later produced their financial modelling report *AnyFire* (LGA 2014) which reported fire and rescue authorities preparing to start the 2014/15 financial year, with on average 33% less in government funding than they had 4 years previously. Whilst Krugman (2012), Blyth (2013) and Schui (2014) chart the policy failure, Stiglitz (2012), O'Hara (2015), Atkinson (2015), Dorling (2015) and others have graphically illustrated some of the actual consequences. This chapter highlights the shifting nature of the governance, accountability and public assurance arrangements for Fire and Rescue services as a key feature or consequence of the period.

This chapter therefore looks at the years between 2010 and 2015, which were a period of long-term austerity and immense uncertainty within UK public services. There was a radical shift in the policy of the central coalition government as it adopted neo-liberal economic policies and imposed significant reductions in public expenditure in response to the recession. Fire and Rescue Services, like all public services throughout the UK, had to adjust to these new financial parameters. However, devolution of powers to Scotland and Wales meant that the organisation and delivery of Fire and Rescue Services diversified between different parts of the union. For example, the governance and structure of the service in Scotland changed radically, whilst arrangements in England hardly altered despite exhortations from the government. On the other hand, accountability, performance management, human resource issues and the services collaboration with key service delivery partners both changed and became more complex throughout the UK. Later chapters discuss these issues in more detail, the changes in both strategic and operational management as well as the consequences for equalities, accountabilities and the relationship of the service to the public. This chapter attempts to give a brief overview to the coalition period to set the scene, survey the organisational landscape and provide a little perspective for these later chapters.

Localism, Dismantling the Improvement Infrastructure and the Strategic Review of the National Framework

In June 2010, the new fire minister announced a 'strategic review' of the fire and rescue sector, the governments' role within it and whether or not a national framework was needed. He acknowledged that the government would have to provide assurance about responding to national emergencies and the adequacy of national and local emergency resilience arrangements. However, he expected FRS to deliver 'more for less', promising greater financial autonomy in the Spending Review in return and announced the abandonment of national diversity targets and national guidance on recruitment and development (DCLG 2010a; Murphy and Greenhalgh 2013); Chaps. 11 and 12 provide a more detailed discussion.

Within 3 months, David Cameron, the Prime Minister, had announced the coming of the Big Society (Cameron 2010) and George Osbourne, the Chancellor, had announced the 'bonfire of the QUANGOs' as part of his emergency budget (HMT 2010). Eric Pickles the Secretary of State for Communities and Local Government confirmed the abolition of the Audit Commission,[2] the termination of Comprehensive Area Assessments (CAA), Local Area Agreements, the National Indicator Set and the 'era of top-down government' (DCLG 2010b, 2010c; Lowndes and Pratchett 2012). The retained firefighter arrangements were, however, promoted, as these were seen as being congruent to both the Big Society and Localism agendas, and the emphasis on prevention, protection and community safety, together with the requirement for Integrated Risk Management Planning (IRMP), also remained.

The LGA had already been promoting sector-led improvement and regulation as a replacement for the Audit Commission's CAA[3] (LGA 2011), and in December 2010, the four *Fire Futures* reports looking at the fire sectors' role, efficiency, accountability and its work with other emergency services was published. The government, in its response to the *Fire Futures* reports in April 2011, made it clear it would only take ideas forward in the light of its emerging policy for public sector reform and the localism agenda (DCLG 2011). This anticipated the forthcoming white paper on public sector reform (Cabinet Office 2011) and the development of sector-led improvement, which both the LGA and the government had supported in their evidence and response to the Select Committee examining the decision to abolish the Audit Commission (House of Commons 2011b).

By the time the select committee published its report in July 2011, the closure of the Audit Commission was a practical inevitability (as acknowledged by the committee itself) as the vast majority of staff had already found alternative employment, although the commission was only formally closed on the 31 March 2015. It is interesting to note that in the final sessions of the select committee hearings, and whilst acknowledging the inevitability of closure, various witnesses[4] were asked directly whether they supported the abolition of the commission including the Chief Fire Officers Association's (CFOA) witness Peter Holland.[5] On behalf of CFOA and the sector, he responded that whilst there were caveats, the commission had on balance been a positive benefit to the service and should be retained and reformed rather than abolished (House of Commons 2011b).

The *Open Public Services White Paper* (Cabinet Office 2011) published on 1 July 2011 was the coalition government's flagship policy for public sector reform. It drew a distinction between three types of public services and the government's intentions towards them:

- Individual or personal services used by people on an individual basis
- Neighbourhood services defined as being provided very locally on a collective rather than an individual basis
- Commissioned services – whether commissioned by central or local government – that cannot be devolved to communities or individuals

Fire and Rescue Services are not mentioned in the white paper, but in the fourth national framework that followed in 2012 (DCLG 2012), it is clear that they are being treated as commissioned services with the Fire and Rescue Authority being the commissioners and the Fire and Rescue Services being the main providers of services.[6]

In commissioned services, there would be separate commissioners and providers, open commissioning and credible independent accreditation of providers. Commissioners are held to account by users and citizens. Providers are held to account through a combination of mutually reinforcing choice (a market of alternative providers), voice (the public as so-called 'armchair' auditors) and transparency mechanisms (more publically available data and information) depending on the service being provided. External audit and inspection would ensure that commissioners and providers both meet acceptable standards and have appropriate financial controls in place.

In 2010, Eric Pickles had also announced the closure of the Government Regional Offices (DCLG 2010d) that formerly hosted the Regional Resilience Forums established by the 2004 Civil Contingencies Act. Regional Offices had previously been tasked to compile and continually review regional risk registers and to co-ordinate the Local Resilience Forums and community risk registers across the regions. They also co-ordinated with the equivalent national resilience arrangements, including the national risk assessment (Cabinet Office 2012, 2015), particularly at times of national or widespread emergencies. The loss of this key part of the infrastructure was particularly exposed in the winter floods of 2013/14 (Murphy 2014) and by the outbreaks of avian influenza ('bird flu') in February 2015.

In summary, the period from May 2010 to July 2012 was dominated by austerity and proposals for reductions in public expenditure, in an attempt to cut the structural deficit and reduce the size of the state. This was accompanied by measures to introduce market mechanisms to reform public services exemplified by the 2012 Health and Social Care Act which led to the extensive (and disastrous) reorganisation of the National Health Service in England. The DCLG was an enthusiastic implementer of these policies and Fire and Rescue Services, like all of the services under the department's portfolio, suffered the consequences.

The National Framework and the Knight Review

The fourth National Framework for Fire and Rescue Services was published in July 2012 with an 'open ended duration'. It was specifically addressed to fire authorities, as commissioners of services rather than the whole service or sector. It was much shorter than its predecessors and covered only England as devolution by this time had transferred responsibility for services in Scotland, Wales and Northern Ireland to their respective parliaments. When dealing with issues and responsibilities arising from the Civil Contingencies Act 2004, the framework is careful to refer to the 'national' roles and responsibilities of both the government and the Fire and Rescue Services. In its desire to avoid saying anything about Scotland, Wales and Northern Ireland, it actually obfuscates the situation.

In his ministerial foreword, Bob Neil summed up the new approach in the following extracts:

> 'In addition to their historic role of putting out fires and coming to our rescue in other emergencies, fire and rescue authorities also work on fire prevention:
>
> * organising home fire safety visits for older people and vulnerable
> * supporting regulatory compliance in the business community and helping minimise the impact of fire on the economy.
>
> There are new challenges. Fire and rescue authorities need to be able to deal with the continuing threat of terrorism, the impact of climate change, and the impacts of an ageing population, against the need to cut the national deficit.
>
> The National Framework will continue to provide an overall strategic direction to fire and rescue authorities, but will not seek to tell them how they should serve their communities. They are free to operate in a way that enables the most efficient delivery of their services. This may include working collaboratively with other fire and rescue authorities, or with other organisations, to improve public safety and cost effectiveness. Ultimately, it is to local communities, not Government, that fire and rescue authorities are accountable'. (DCLG 2012, p. 6)

Introducing the framework in July 2012 was one of the final acts that Bob Neil undertook in government as, after the summer recess, he was replaced in September 2012 by Brandon Lewis MP.

Delivery and Performance: Sector Led Improvement, Fire Peer Challenge and Operational Assessments

As mentioned above, the new coalition and the Local Government Association were committed to a sector-led improvement and regulatory system since the 2010 election, with local government and DCLG in the vanguard. The dismantling of the previous system between 2010 and 2012 compelled both the local government sector and the fire and rescue sector to take more responsibility for their own regulation and performance. Chapter 5 evaluates the effectiveness of fire peer challenge and the operational assessment of Fire and Rescue Services, the key elements of the sector's new approach to performance improvement, whilst Chaps. 13 and 14 examine some of these issues in Scotland and Wales from a devolved government perspective.

The next part of this chapter looks at the 'improved' public assurance, accountability and transparency arrangements that were supposed to be the purpose and hallmark of the new arrangements for commissioned services as envisioned by the coalition governments' public service reform programme introduced by the Open Public Services White Paper and delivered under the 2012 National Framework. At the time of writing, these remain in place although, as explained in Chap. 17, the central government responsibility for Fire and Rescue Services in England was transferred back to the Home Office in January 2016, and legislative proposals for the transfer of local governance, policy and delivery to elected local mayors or police and crime commissioners are well advanced.[7]

Public and Stakeholder Assurance Arrangements Between 2010 and 2015[8]

The development of the public assurance regime in Fire and Rescue Services, under the Conservative-led coalition government (which includes the performance management arrangements discussed in more detail in Chap. 5 and accountability arrangements in Chaps. 8, 13, 14 and 15 require four interrelated yet independent key areas to be examined. These areas collectively give an indication of the quality, quantity, scope and maturity of the prevailing arrangements for public and stakeholder assurance. Each is a necessary element of the assurance landscape, but each on its own is insufficient to provide an overall judgement.

The following analysis could be criticised for overemphasising horizontal and top-down assurance, but as one of the prime objectives of the nation state is to protect its citizens, emergency (and security) services have historically and predominantly been scrutinised hierarchically and vertically. This has been the case within the UK in the past, with the prime responsibility falling to the national government. It is almost certain that the devolution of police, fire and ambulance services to Scotland, Wales and Northern Ireland, and the ongoing devolution of police and fire service to elected mayors, and police and crime commissioners will alter these responsibilities and relationships in the future. The four key factors are:

(a) The adequacy of the accountability and transparency arrangements in place for the service, at national and local levels
(b) The development and maturity of the data and intelligence that forms the evidential base for the development and deployment of policy and practice within the service

(c) The adequacy of the service's governance, its leadership and the extent of the strategic alignment within the service, and with its key partners such as local government, ambulance and police services

(d) The adequacy of public reporting, public scrutiny and the arrangements for intervention in the event of failing or significantly underperforming delivery

Accountability and Transparency

Hood's (2010) seminal paper examined the complex interrelationships between accountability and transparency and rhetorically likened them to Siamese twins, matching parts or an awkward couple. He appreciated that they had a complicated overlapping relationship to one another, which distinguished him from the Secretary of State Eric Pickles, who repeatedly sought to claim that greater transparency was the same as greater accountability (DCLG 2012).[9]

The secretary of state was, however, accountable to parliament for the overall stewardship of Fire and Rescue Services in England between 2010 and 2015. The DCLG's accounting officer aka, the permanent secretary, was accountable to parliament for the stewardship of resources allocated via DCLG to the 46 Fire and Rescue Authorities (FRAs). The accounting officer provides assurance to parliament that grants made by the DCLG are properly accounted for by Fire and Rescue Autorities (FRA) and should ensure regularity, propriety and value for money or, if necessary, advise the secretary of state on the use of intervention powers.

The roles and responsibilities of the local FRA are contained in the third Fire and Rescue National Framework for England (DCLG 2012) published in July 2012. Individual FRAs oversee the policy and service delivery of a Fire and Rescue Service. The chief fire officer (CFO) is responsible for the day-to-day command of the FRS and is accountable to the FRA.

Financial provision for fire and rescue is provided through the Local Government Departmental Expenditure Limit (DEL); a local share of business rates under the rates retention scheme, a levy on Council Tax, and fees and charges from services such as training.

Financial controls includes clear responsibilities around expenditure, financial duties and rules for prudence in spending, internal checks for compliance and external checks by an independent auditor.

FRAs are currently subject to the auditing and accounting regime introduced by the Local Audit and Accountability Act 2014, which repealed the Audit Commission Act 1998. This gives local bodies freedom to appoint their own auditors and manage their own audit arrangements. The new audit framework reflects the regulatory roles found in the Companies sector. The NAO has produced the code of practice and supporting guidelines and enhanced existing programmes of value for money examinations to carry out a small number of studies to take in local delivery. In November 2015, the NAO produced both a Local Government Report *Financial stability of fire and rescue services* and a Value for Money Study *Variation in spending by fire and rescue authorities 2011–12 to 2013–14* (NAO 2015a, 2015b).

Since 2010, the FRS performance management regime, including arrangements for assessing value for money, have, in practice, been focussed around the LGA sector-led improvement approach, which is discussed in more detail in Chap. 5. The former independent Her Majesty's Fire Service Inspectorate was decommissioned in 2007, although the NAO report mentioned above and the subsequent Public Accounts Committee hearings based on the report have called for its restitution. England and Wales are unusual as countries in being without independent fire inspectorates (in Scotland and Northern Ireland the role was retained). The chief fire service advisor (CFSA) role was created in 2007 and is often mistaken for Her Majesty's Inspectorate. The CFSA is a civil servant subject to the civil service code and answerable to the department the DCLG between 2010 and 2015 and the Home Office since 2016.

The Local Authority (Executive Arrangements) (Meetings and Access to Information) (England) Regulations 2012 were intended to introduce greater transparency and openness into council meetings and also apply to FRAs. Members of the public can only be refused admission in limited circumstances, and they must be able to access documents that relate to meetings and executive decisions.

DCLG's *Code of Recommended Practice on Data Transparency*, also known as the *Local Government Transparency Code 2014* also applies to the FRA. As such, it lists a range of datasets that FRSs must make available to the public. These include publication of annual accounts and each line of spending worth over £500. It also comprises senior employee salaries, including the officer's name (with consent), job description, responsibilities, budgets and number of staff. In addition, it includes councillor allowances and expenses, copies of contracts and tenders, and grants to the voluntary and social enterprise sectors. Furthermore, it includes policies, performance and external audit, and covers key inspections and key indicators on fiscal and financial position.

Evidence, Information and the Capacity to Interrogate and Analyse

A coalition government proposal to outsource the collection, analysis and reporting of the government's Fire Service Statistics by DCLG in 2013 met with little enthusiasm from potential providers and has not yet been implemented. The governments 'Fire statistics', together with financial and performance databases from CFOA and CIPFA, allow for investigation and analysis of expenditure and other performance information, although the latter two are only available to subscribers.

In practice, the collection, analysis, availability, transparency and interrogation of fire data, particularly performance data by independent researchers, have become increasingly difficult since 2010. This is due, in part, to the demise of the Audit

Commission, which collected and published national performance statistics and made them publicly available on interactive websites. The Commissions' national reports have been lodged in the National Archives but neither the local reports nor the data on the interactive websites are any longer available.

The Audit Commission produced 28 national reports relating specifically to fire and rescue management between 1983 and 2010, and numerous others with direct and indirect relevance. This loss of capacity has only been partially compensated for by operational research capacity and capability at the NAO, but this is much smaller and NAO databases are not interactive. Historically, there has been little independent academic research capacity in the management of fire and rescue (Wankheda and Murphy 2012).

The Fire Peer Challenge and Operational Assessment (see Chap. 5), commissioned by all 46 FRSs in England and Wales or the Fire Authorities response to the reviews were initially published on the Local Governments Association website although they were withdrawn by the LGA in 2015 and only a minority are available on Authority websites.

Governance Leadership and Strategic Alignment

As explained in Chap. 2, the years immediately before and after the turn of the twenty-first century were characterised by poor governance, fragmented leadership and a lack of strategic alignment at local and national levels (Bain et al. 2002). These problems were exacerbated by the national firefighters' strike which lasted over 5 years from 1998 to 2003. Between 2003 and 2010, central and local government, local FRSs, CFOA and the Audit Commission sought to re-establish collective sector leadership and facilitate performance improvement, innovation and service delivery.

The Fire and Rescue Act 2004 and the Civil Contingencies Act 2004 were the start of a period of gradual acceptance and engagement (see Chap. 3). This process was characterised by increasing strategic alignment through joined-up policy and delivery, improved performance management, and investment in infrastructure and system support. Although the development of tools, techniques, systems and interventions were always some way behind developments in the equivalent health and local government regimes, they were rapidly progressing and generally considered to be ahead of FRSs worldwide. For example, the Integrated Risk Management Planning (IRMP) process received international recognition with Scotland (Scottish Fire and Rescue Service 2013), Ireland (National Directorate for Fire and Emergency Services 2012), Europe, Australia, New Zealand, Canada and others, gradually adopting similar approaches or parts of the process.

Since 2010, this collective leadership has fragmented, with significant loss of capacity and coherence, accompanied by a loss of collective vision, thereby compromising strategic alignment (Murphy 2015; NAO 2015a, NAOb). The coalition government significantly reduced its own role, as demonstrated in the fourth National

Framework (DCLG 2012, Brown 2014). As in previous periods of the FRS's history (Raynsford 2016), leadership and collective responsibility has largely been left to CFOA, and there is a clear risk to individual and collective aspirations for efficiency and value for money (Knight 2013; NAO 2015a, NAO 2015b). Although the LGA has offered a Financial Health Check (LGA 2013) under their sector-led improvement programme since 2013 (LGA 2014), there is no evidence that this has been embraced or had an impact in FRSs. In practice, FRSs (and FRAs) in England have been driven by the theory and practice of short-term cutback management throughout the period of the coalition government.

Fire services deal with short and long-term emergencies with other blue light services on a day-to-day basis. The FRA's role is to finance and equip the response to incidents and emergencies and to allow the service to collaborate and deliver strategic and operational efficiencies. It is the Local Resilience Forums that make inter-agency operational response efficient and effective. The emergency services generally, including FRSs, have very mature efficient and effective cross-organisational emergency planning, resilience and interoperability capability at an operational response level, and this has improved continually since modern emergency services were established after the Second World War. The national interoperability has similarly improved since the Civil Contingencies Act in 2004; however, regional planning, coordination and response capacity was lost when Regional Risk Registers, Regional Resilience Forums and Regional Government Officers were closed in 2012.

Reporting Scrutiny and Intervention

The chief fire and rescue advisor provides strategic advice and guidance to ministers, civil servants and FRAs on the structure, organisation and performance of FRAs and FRSs, although he has no reporting obligations to parliament or to the public other than through the DCLG. Apart from annual financial reporting, individual FRSs have no reporting responsibilities, other than statistical returns to parliament, DCLG, the secretary of state or other regulators or agencies. Their financial reporting responsibilities are enshrined in the Local Audit and Accountability Act 2014.

The Open Government White Paper (Cabinet Office 2011) and the third National Framework for England (DCLG 2012) clearly differentiated the responsibilities of FRAs and FRSs along the 'commissioner provider' split, and scrutiny is largely exercised at the local level through local government structures, regulations and practices. However, there is no demonstrable evidence that this has made any significant impact in practice and no discernible impact on either the amount or quality of scrutiny by FRAs.

The relevant inter-agency and collaborative working arrangements are 'horizontally' scrutinised in Local Resilience Forums that emerged out of long-standing local emergency planning groups and Health and Wellbeing Boards that are of relatively recent origin and therefore untested in their 'scrutiny' role, and community safety partnerships.

In terms of expenditure and budgeting, all FRSs are able to benchmark through CIPFA's interactive financial database and its interrogative tools. In terms of external scrutiny, however, the FRAs and FRSs have considerable discretion to determine what is reported to the public, when and in what detail. As a result, their reports and the data behind them are variable and not particularly useful for the purposes of conducting meaningful comparisons across organisations and scrutinising their activities as Murphy et al. (2012) found in a previous survey for Nottinghamshire FRS and more recently (Ferry and Murphy 2015) for the NAO.

FRAs and FRSs are subject to the duty of Best Value, and the secretary of state for DCLG has broad intervention powers conferred by the Local Government Act 1999 and the Fire and Rescue Services Act 2004. Section 28 of the latter Act provides powers to obtain information or to take action in any circumstances where the central government may wish to have an investigation or assessment. This could include a major fire incident investigation or where there are serious concerns regarding the discharging of their functions or even corporate failure. Sections 22 and 23 allow the secretary of state to intervene if there is a risk that an FRA/FRS will fail, provided they consult and demonstrate why this risk is imminent or serious. The secretary of state is required to have regard to the updated *Protocol on government intervention action on fire and rescue authorities in England* (DCLG 2013) although this has not been used to date. As explained in more detail in this chapter, the central government's expectation is that sector partners will provide initial support. In other words, ministers would only intervene in the most serious of failures, or if sector support is refused or incapable of turning around the underperformance.

Summary

A report commissioned by the NAO from Ferry and Murphy (2015) assessed the quality and effectiveness of public assurance being provided across locally delivered public services including Fire and Rescue Services. This found that accountability and transparency were generally poorer in 2015 than it was in 2010. The performance management regime was fragmenting, the evidence base diminishing and there had been a significant loss of capacity and capability in the improvement infrastructure and support available to fire services. Major capital funding arrangements (principally the Public Finance Initiative) remained inflexible and expensive, and financial and resource planning was generally short term and conformance dominated. As Knight (2013) had found earlier, and the NAO later suspected (NAO 2015a, 2015b), potential inter-agency efficiency gains were not being captured still less maximised.

In an attempt to illustrate the historical and sector changes and the relative positions of the various services, Ferry and Murphy produced a series of diagrams which

showed the level of public assurance and the likely risk to achieving value for money
(as defined in traditional terms in relation to economy, efficiency and effectiveness).
The relevant diagrams for Fire and Rescue Services are reproduced below. A 'green'
rating represented best available practice plus known achievable potential improvements as existing in 2010. The (by then) new Conservative governments' immediate
response was to transfer responsibility back to the Home Office in January 2016.
This period will be discussed later in Chap. 17.

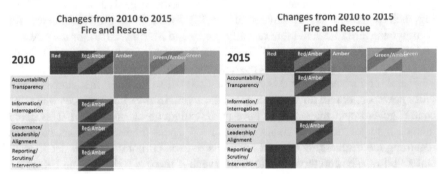

Notes

1. There is now an academic journal entitled *Resilience Journal*.
2. This was the first of 15 budgets delivered by the Chancellor between 2010 and
   2016, before his dismissal in July 2016.
3. There had been a leak and considerable press coverage about the potential abolition of Audit Commission prior to this official statement.
4. By the end of 13 years of new Labour administration, the conservatives overwhelmingly controlled the LGA and dominated the response to the Conservative-
   led coalition's policy and the invited submissions and appearances at the DCLG
   Select Committee hearings.
5. Later to become the second chief fire adviser to the DCLG. The first was Sir Ken
   Knight.
6. Prior to the fourth national framework, government legislation and guidance normally referred to services or to authorities and services collectively – for the first
   time this framework was exclusively addressed to FRAs. The change was also
   meant to facilitate the private sector in the potential supply of services to
   authorities.
7. At the time of writing the Crime and Policing Bill, which will facilitate Police
   and Crime Commissioners or Elected Mayors assuming responsibility for the
   governance of FRSs, had reached its third reading in parliament. This is discussed in more detail in Chap. 17.
8. The remaining parts of this chapter draw heavily on reports by the authors commissioned by the NAO. The first was commissioned and (part) funded by the

NAO, and any errors or omissions are the responsibility of the authors. The NAO does not necessarily endorse the findings of the work.

9. This statement from the secretary of state is no longer available and was later corrected and 'updated' on the government's websites on 8 May 2015 (DCLG 2015a, b).

References

Atkinson, A. (2015). *Inequality: What can be done?* Cambridge Mass: Harvard University Press.

Audit Commission. (2008). *Crunch time: The impact of the economic downturn on local government finances*. London: Audit Commission.

Audit Commission. (2009). *When it comes to the crunch: How councils are responding to the recession*. London: Audit Commission.

Audit Commission. (2010). *Surviving the crunch: Local finances in the recession and beyond*. London: Audit Commission.

Barbera, C., Jones, M., Saliterer, I., & Steccolini, I. (2014). European local authorities' financial resilience in the face of austerity: A comparison across Austria, Italy and England. International Conference on Next Steps for Public Administration in Theory and Practice: Sun Yat-Sen University, Guangzhou, China, Nov 2014.

Bain, G., Lyons, M., & Young, M. (2002). *The future of the Fire Service:reducing risks, saving lives: the independent review of the Fire Service*. London: TSO.

Blyth, M. (2013). *Austerity. The history of a dangerous idea*. Oxford: Oxford University Press.

Brown, L. (2014). *The future of fire and rescue services in England – A survey for shadow minister Lyn Brown MP*. London: House of Commons.

Cabinet Office. (2011). *Open public services white paper*. London: Cabinet Office.

Cabinet Office. (2012). *Chapter 16 collaboration and co-operation between local resilience forums in England revision to emergency preparedness*. London: TSO.

Cabinet Office. (2015). *National Risk Register of Civil Emergencies 2015 edition*. London: TSO.

Cameron, D. (2010). *Big society speech*. London: Cabinet Office.

Department of Communities and Local Government. (2010a). *Leading a lean and efficient fire and rescue service*, fire minister bob Neill's speech to fire and rescue 2010 conference, Harrogate, England.

Department of Communities and Local Government. (2010b). *Eric pickles to disband audit commission in new era of town hall transparency*. Announcement as a news item 25th June 2010 that the Secretary of State had written instructing the Audit Commission to terminate CAA. Available at https://www.gov.uk/government/news/eric-pickles-to-disband-audit-commission-in-new-era-of-town-hall-transparency.

Department of Communities and Local Government. (2010c). *Local Government Accountability*. Written Statement to Parliament. 13th Oct 2010. Available at https://www.gov.uk/government/speeches/local-government-accountability--2.

Department of Communities and Local Government. (2010d). *Pickles outlines plans to abolish regional government* Announcement as a news item 22nd July 2010. Available at https://www.gov.uk/government/news/pickles-outlines-plans-to-abolish-regional-government.

Department of Communities and Local Government. (2011). *Fire Futures reports government response*. London: DCLG.

Department of Communities and Local Government. (2012). *Local council transparency and accountability*. London: TSO.

Department of Communities and Local Government. (2013). *Protocol on government intervention action on fire and rescue authorities in England*. London: DCLG.

Department of Communities and Local Government. (2015a). 2010 to 2015 government policy: Local council transparency and accountability as updated 8th May 2015. Available at https://www.gov.uk/government/publications/2010-to-2015-government-policy-local-council-transparency-and-accountability

Department of Communities and Local Government. (2015b). *Fire and rescue; Operational Statistics Bulletin for England 2014–2015*. London: TSO.

Dorling, D. (2015). *Injustice: Why social inequality still persists* (Revised ed., p. 484). Bristol: Policy Press.

Ferry, L., & Murphy, P. (2015). Financial sustainability, accountability and transparency across local public service bodies in England under austerity. Report to National Audit Office. Nottingham: Nottingham Trent University.

Her Majesty's Treasury. (2010). *Budget June 2010*. (Emergency Budget) London: HMT.

Hood, C. (2010). Accountability and transparency: Siamese twins, matching parts or awkward couple? *West European Politics, 33*(5), 989–1009.

House of Commons. (2011b). *Select committee: Audit and inspection of local authorities – communities and local government committee 4th report*. Norwich: TSO.

Knight, K., Sir. (2013). *Sir Ken Knights's independent review of efficiency and operations in fire and rescue authorities in England*. London: DCLG.

Krugman, P. (2012). *End this depression now*. New York: Norton.

Local Government Association. (2011). *Taking the lead: self-regulation and improvement in local government*. London: LGA.

Local Government Association. (2013). *A guide to our sectot-led improvement offer for finance*. London: LGA.

Local Government Association. (2014). *AnyFire the future funding outlook for fire and rescue authorities*. London: LGA.

Local Government Association. (2015). *Taking stock: Where next with sector-led improvement?* London: LGA.

Lowndes, V., & McCaughie, K. (2013). Weathering the perfect storm? Austerity and institutional resilience in local government. *Policy & Politics, 41*(4), 534–549.

Lowndes, V., & Pratchett, L. (2012). Local Governance under the Coalition Government: Austerity, Localism and the 'Big Society'. *Local Government Studies, 38*(1), 21–40.

Murphy, P. (2014). Flood response hit by regional austerity cuts. London: The Conversation Media Group UK.

Murphy, P. (2015). *Briefing note on Financial sustainability offire and rescue services – value for money report for the NAO*. London: National Audit Office.

Murphy, P., & Greenhalgh, K. (2013). Performance management in fire and rescue services. *Public Money & Management, 33*(3), 225–232.

Murphy, P., Greenhalgh, K., & Parkin, C. (2012). Fire and rescue service configuration: a case study in Nottinghamshire. *International Journal of Emergency Services, 1*(2), 182–189.

National Audit Office. (2015a). Department for communities and local government; Financial stability of fire and rescue services. HC 491 London: NAO.

National Audit Office. (2015b). *Variation in spending by fire and rescue authorities 2011–12 to 2013–14*. London: NAO.

National Directorate for Fire and Emergency Services. (2012). *Keeping communities safe – a framework for fire safety in Ireland*. Dublin: Department of Environment, Community and Local Government.

O'Hara, M. (2015). *Austerity bites: A journey to the sharp end of cuts in the UK*. Bristol: Bristol Policy Press.

Raynsford, N. (2016). *Substance not spin: An insider's view of success and failure in government*. Bristol: Policy Press.

Schui, F. (2014). *Austerity. The great failure*. New Haven: Yale University Press.

Scottish Fire and Rescue Services. (2013). *Fire and rescue framework for Scotland 2013*. Edinburgh, The Scottish Government. ISBN: 9781782564270.

Steccolini, I., Guarini, E., Barbera, C., & Jones, M. (2014). Financial resilience in local authorities: An exploration of Anglo-Italian experiences. IRSPM 2014: D1 Special Interest Group: Accounting and Accountability, Ottawa.

Stiglitz, J. (2012). *The price of inequality: How Today's divided Society endangers our future*. New York: Norton.

Walker, A. (2015). *Resilience in practice*. London: Local Government Information Unit.

Wankhade, P., & Murphy, P. (2012). Bridging the theory and practice gap in emergency services research: the case for a new journal. *International Journal of Emergency Services, 1*(1), 4–9.

Dr. Laurence Ferry PhD (Warwick), BA (Hons) 1st Class, FCPFA, SFHEA, PACAPL is an Professor in Accounting at Durham University Business School. He earned his PhD from the Warwick Business School and is a qualified accountant, Fellow of the Chartered Institute of Public Finance and Accountancy (FCPFA) and Senior Fellow of the Higher Education Academy (SFHEA). His research, teaching and consulting covers accounting and accountability with a specific focus on the public sector where he is a recognised international expert in public sector accounting and accountability having dealt with 30 countries.

Chapter 5
Peer Challenge: A Sector-Led Approach to Performance Improvement in Fire and Rescue Services

James Downe, Steve Martin, and Heike Doering

Introduction

Fire and rescue services (FRSs) have been subject to a range of different performance improvement regimes in recent years including Best Value, Comprehensive Performance Assessment (CPA) and Comprehensive Area Assessment (CAA). These have been criticised for being top-down, costly, not providing significant 'added-value' and focusing upon corporate processes rather than operational performance. The abolition of the Audit Commission, which oversaw these regimes, allowed the sector to take greater responsibility for its own regulation and performance. This chapter evaluates the effectiveness of fire peer challenge and the operational assessment (OpA), which form important elements of the sector's current approach to performance improvement and public assurance.

Assessing the Performance of Fire and Rescue Services in England

The current fire peer challenge approach comprises a number of elements of previous performance regimes, so a brief summary provides important context (see Murphy and Greenhalgh (2013a) for a detailed analysis of regimes used in fire and rescue services). In 1999, the Local Government Act included Fire and Rescue Services (FRSs) together with local authorities in the Best Value regime. As a result, continuous improvement of their services became a statutory requirement. The core

J. Downe (✉) • S. Martin • H. Doering
Cardiff Business School, Cardiff University, Cardiff, UK
e-mail: downej@cardiff.ac.uk

© Springer International Publishing AG 2018
P. Murphy, K. Greenhalgh (eds.), *Fire and Rescue Services*,
DOI 10.1007/978-3-319-62155-5_5

principles of the Best Value approach were the introduction of national performance indicators and increased attention to organisational rather than simply operational performance. These principles were supposed to facilitate the 'modernisation' not just of the Fire and Rescue Service, but the wider local public service. Part of this modernisation agenda was a reordering of employment relations in FRSs, which sparked a prolonged dispute within the sector (Andrews 2010). This dispute was finally resolved through the Bain Review of 2002, but little progress was made in terms of 'reforming' FRSs along new public management lines until the Fire and Rescue Service Act of 2004.

This Act brought a renewed emphasis on performance management through a new CPA (2002–2008). This focused on specified corporate areas as well as performance against national indicators, but also introduced a reorientation of aims and objectives of FRSs. The Act placed the new duty of prevention and the management of risk to life (rather than property) at the centre for FRSs (Andrews 2010). This reorientation coupled with a plethora of key performance indicators and lack of focus on operational assessment (Murphy and Jones 2016) led to criticism of CPA. The CAA regime (2008–2010) focused on the collective achievement of public service outcomes in a given local authority, but was quickly abolished by the coalition government which wanted to reduce the cost of centralised performance regimes and devolve responsibility for improvement to lower levels. As a result, national performance indicators were removed and sector organisations stepped into the regulatory void left by the abolition of the Audit Commission.

Fire Peer Challenge

Fire peer challenge was designed by the Local Government Association (LGA) in partnership with the Chief Fire Officers Association (CFOA). It builds on previous experiences of peer challenge and is an important element of its sector-led approach to improvement. The process complements and is integrated with the industry standard Operational Assessment Toolkit (OpA). It emphasises that fire services are responsible for their own performance and is underpinned by three key design principles:

- Stronger local accountability leads to further improvement.
- Fire and Rescue Services have a sense of collective responsibility for performance in the sector as a whole.
- The LGA's role is to help FRSs by providing the necessary support.

Fire peer challenges are managed and delivered by the sector for the sector and each fire service is offered a peer challenge once every three years. This chapter examines the effectiveness of the fire peer challenge methodology and the Operational Assessment Toolkit and the overall impact of fire peer challenges in helping the sector with self-monitoring and improvement.

Methods

The chapter is based on a series of in-depth, semi-structured interviews with the Chair, chief fire officer (CFO) and the officer who was most closely involved in the fire peer challenge in a sample of ten[1] fire and rescue services. The case studies included different types of services (county, combined and metropolitan fire authorities) and two (Surrey and West Yorkshire) that had helped pilot OpA and fire peer challenge. Interviews were conducted by phone on a non-attributable basis using a topic guide that covered the key aspects of the process and its impacts. Each interview was recorded and the key points noted in contemporaneous notes.

We also conducted an online survey of senior officers and councillors in each of the FRSs that had completed a fire peer challenge by the time of the study. The survey examined the impact that fire peer challenge had in helping the sector with self-monitoring and improvement. We received 24 completed surveys from 17 (74%) fire authorities[2] who had undertaken OpA and fire peer challenge.

The Operational Assessment

The Operational Assessment (OpA) covers seven key assessment areas (community risk management, prevention, protection, response, health and safety, training and development, call management and incident support) and fire services saw it as a very important contributor to service improvement. The process helped officers to ensure that the service is working well operationally and provided councillors with valuable reassurance on performance.

All of the case studies took the OpA process very seriously and devoted a lot of time to preparing for it as it complemented and informed the focus of the peer challenge. As one interviewee explained:

> A robust self-assessment provided a process for the team to probe and it made the challenge rounded.

There were concerns, however, that it would be possible for fire services to manage the OpA in order to obtain a favourable report. None of interviewees admitted to this kind of 'gaming', but one officer explained that:

> There is an opportunity to put all your good stuff into the OpA and leave out your weaknesses. I'm sure that some fire services follow this strategy.

Nearly all survey respondents (96%) agreed that the OpA had helped them to undertake an honest appraisal of their performance. The overwhelming view from

---

[1] Bedfordshire and Luton FRS, Cheshire FRS, Cornwall FRS, Hampshire FRS, Hertfordshire FRS, Merseyside FRS, Staffordshire FRS, Surrey FRS, West Yorkshire FRS, Wiltshire FRS.

[2] The survey used a five-point Likert scale. For ease of reporting, we have grouped the 4 = 'tend to agree' and 5 = 'strongly agree' into agree.

interviewees was that the sector as a whole has matured in recent years to the point where services are much more willing to identify areas for improvement and keen to use OpA as a learning process, rather than trying to impress others. One CFO explained that:

> It's all about having the confidence to admit weaknesses and it doesn't hurt to say we need to be better here.

There is potential for the OpA to focus more upon the quality and effectiveness of a service, rather than relying on process measures and to use performance measures to examine how services compare with each other. In this way, it could contribute to the building of a transparent evidence base to ensure robustness of the process and facilitate public assurance (Murphy and Greenhalgh 2014).

The Process

The CFOA and the LGA have documented how the process works and the roles and responsibilities of each party. This guidance is helpful in enabling services to scope the challenge, set clear expectations and make sure all the necessary preparations are made. As it is not possible for peer challenge to cover all of the areas included in the OpA in sufficient depth, each service can tailor the process to their own particular needs. The focus of the challenge was often determined by a service's recent history of performance. For example, services with a history of performance problems saw the peer challenge as an opportunity to receive an independent review of their improvement journey. At the other end of the performance spectrum, services hoped it would enable them to stay at the leading edge. As one interviewee put it:

> We have the ambition to be the best fire and rescue service. Therefore, we are almost constantly looking at how we can improve, how we can do better.

The aim of the OpA and fire peer challenge is to be forward-looking. In contrast to previous inspection processes, fire peer challenge starts from a position where services have already identified the issues where they would most value assistance. These issues are examined during the peer challenge along with all the key assessment areas. Peer challenge teams approached their task as 'critical friends' as well as providing ideas and 'notable practice' on how to improve.

The success of the peer challenge depends very much on how a service approaches it. To be effective, it requires honesty, openness and a willingness to learn. One councillor explained that he:

> Learnt through previous inspection processes that if you tell the truth, you learn more, so let's get better ideas from others.

The process was seen by respondents as one designed to help them. This meant that staff engaged positively with the process and tried to get the most out of it. As one interviewee told us:

We've identified these issues. We want you to have a look at them...Give us some fresh, new ideas, some things that you know have worked elsewhere or are being tried elsewhere and actually give us this check of, 'I know you're doing this but have you thought of doing that?'

Preparation for the peer challenge is important as this is the service's investment in the process. We found that the amount of time and resource invested varied significantly between services. One service spent about 7–8 months preparing for the challenge and had written a long and detailed self-assessment. Other services had decided to adopt what they described as a 'lighter touch' approach. For example, in one case the chief fire officer had set a limit of 20 pages for the self-assessment so that it did not take too much time and resource.

It is important that the LGA and CFOA should continue to work with fire and rescue services to scope the challenge carefully so that services decide whether they would like the focus to be broad and shallow or narrow and deep. They should also consider introducing more flexibility within the process so that there is variation on how long a team spends on site which is determined by the content of the OpA and the specific focus for the challenge.

The Team

The fire peer challenge process stands and falls by the quality of the team. Our evidence suggests that the expertise and experience of team members has been very strong. Peers were described as being very capable and to have conducted the challenge in a professional manner. Most services felt that the team that had visited them had the right balance of expertise including front-line operational experience, capable senior fire officers and an experienced councillor. Fire service professionals appreciated the fact that team members had experience of working in/overseeing fire and rescue services. We were told, for example, that a chief fire officer leading a team would be able to distinguish the routine complaints which happen everywhere from genuine concerns. This contrasts with Audit Commission inspectors who often had no first-hand expertise in the sector and might have taken everything at face value.

While interviewees reported that challenge teams were well prepared, insightful and got to grips with the issues very quickly, there were a few instances where team members were seen as relatively new to the process and still finding their feet. Some team members were said to have problems understanding different governance arrangements (e.g. where a fire service sits within a council directorate which has wider responsibilities beyond fire). It is important, therefore, that peers understand how different organisational structures work and take the opportunity to explore and if necessary challenge the evidence base for a course of action.

Three-quarters of survey respondents agreed that their service had a clear idea of who it wanted to form the fire peer challenge team and many had worked with the LGA to identify an appropriate team leader. This makes sense because the relationship between the team leader and the chief fire officer is an important one:

> We did not want a CFO from a small rural shire. We have a very diverse community so we
> wanted someone on the team who understood the community we serve.

Another service had a chief fire officer from a service with different governance arrangements to their own because they saw some value in learning from someone with a different background.

The Knight Review concluded that 'for the process to be meaningful and inspire confidence, services should not be able to continue to choose the review team' (2013: 65). We understand this concern and the public perception that the relationship between the service and challenge team may be seen as too 'cosy'. It was an issue that was highlighted by several interviewees. For example, one chief fire officer told us that:

> The ability to select the team potentially undermines the objectivity of fire challenge.

However, if the leader of the challenge is not the right fit for the service, it is likely to lead to frustration and a lack of understanding. In most cases, the selection of the team was an iterative process where names were provided by the LGA and fire and rescue services offered their views on suitability. We believe that the LGA should continue to discuss the composition of the team with the service and then work to deliver the most appropriate team for each peer challenge. It is also important to recognise the important role played by the LGA manager in being the independent steward for the process. They bring expert knowledge from experiences conducting other challenges and help to counterbalance any accusations about the closeness of the service to the team.

The style of the team is also important in helping to drive change. Interviewees reported that teams were generally open in their approach and there were good team dynamics and extensive discussions amongst the team where they tried to triangulate information. One interviewee summarised by saying that:

> Peer challenge works best if there is humility: humility in learning from others…If there is
> ever a problem, then this is because people give advice without this humility attached to it.

While there have been successful examples where peers from outside the fire sector have joined the team, the process could be improved by having wider representation from outside the fire services. There was strong support across our case studies for widening the expertise within teams where this was appropriate to the focus of the challenge. Interviewees mentioned the police and representatives from the private and voluntary sector. The advantage of 'outsiders' is that they come without preconceived ideas of how the fire service should operate and can bring new ideas that have the potential to quicken the pace of improvement. At the same time, they can provide crucial independence to the process while maintaining the focus on a sector-driven approach to improvement compared to centrally driven performance regimes (Murphy and Greenhalgh 2014).

Reporting

The peer team produce a report at the end of the process which outlines their findings and recommendations for improvement. Nearly all survey respondents (96%) said that the report provided a fair reflection of the organisation's strengths and areas for improvement. Three-quarters agreed that the report was based on strong evidence.

Interviewees were happy with the tone of reports and described them as being 'good', 'pretty balanced', 'positive and helpful' and most were content with the level of detail in the report. However, nearly a third of officers (30%) suggested that the report could have been more challenging. In some of the case studies, we were told that the meeting at the end of the challenge often provided challenging feedback but the written report pulled its punches. One interviewee described the report as being:

Too short, too light and did not provide enough on value for money.

Another felt that:

The report was too generic, too broad brush, too loose. You could take [Name of service] off the front of the report and replace it by any other fire service.

It is important that the reports are robust and comprehensive and reflect the feedback provided at the end of the visit.

Almost all respondents (96%) said that the report did not contain any surprises. This may raise a question about the 'value-added' provided by the process, although it can also be argued that if a fire service is self-aware and conducted a thorough OpA, then there should be no surprises. As one officer said:

There was nothing surprising in the report. I would have been horrified if there was.

Interviewees reported that there was a significant amount of learning which takes place beyond the report through informal discussions. This was seen by some as being more valuable than the formal report as it was an opportunity to pick the brains of a good quality team and to talk 'off-record' as well as to network. For example, one service was considering building new fire stations and changing how they staff them. Members of the team had recently been through this change and were able to pass on their experiences.

Our case studies revealed that the team often provided examples of good practice along the lines of 'why not look at this and see if you can learn from this good practice'? This stops the service wasting months of officer time researching for information when a FRS has already implemented something successfully. The majority felt that more examples of good practice could be shared during the fire peer challenge but also after the process.

Most respondents (92%) agreed that their service had developed an action plan in response to the report. Those which had not done so had picked out the main issues from the report and put them into their service plan. This result compares very favourably with local councils that have been through a similar process called corporate peer challenge. There is no formal opportunity to have a follow-up visit within the fire peer challenge process, although we did hear of a few examples of continuing contact. In one service, a member peer was asked to return and present the report to the whole authority. In another, a two-day 'away-day' was set up so that two services could discuss different approaches to officer-member working and performance management.

We found mixed responses on the idea of a follow-up visit. For some, this was unnecessary as it is up to the service to determine what to take forward and when. This was supported by an interviewee who suggested that:

The peer challenge supports the findings of the self-assessment and as part of the process of self-discovery leading to continuous improvement there is no further need for contact.

Each service has senior managers who should be able to respond to issues within the report as well as councillors scrutinising performance. A follow-up visit would require further investment in time by members of the peer challenge team.

A number of fire services thought that a follow-up visit could have significant benefits. It would not be necessary for all services but a light-touch visit could help to ensure that areas for consideration were implemented. As one officer admitted:

> Since the fire peer challenge, action and effort relating to the identified areas of improvement has diminished and a follow-up would provide more focus.

The LGA and CFOA should formalise the current arrangements so that services may receive additional support from members of the peer challenge team where there is demand and resource capacity.

Services have taken different approaches to sharing the findings. In one, staff gathered to hear the messages from the team first-hand. Their one disappointment was not getting a score ('fair' or 'good') on the final slide. In another service, the report was shared with senior staff only, but the chief fire officer has used the headline findings as part of two briefings to staff.

The Knight Review suggested that 'Review reports should be published together with an action plan as a matter of course' (2013: 65). To date, all fire and rescue authorities have published the report on their website and we believe it is important that this continues. Just over half have communicated the report with partners or to residents (56%). While the process is not explicitly aimed at providing reassurance to the public, the report can help those members of the public interested in understanding the key issues facing the organisation, but is not sufficient on its own to provide public confidence (Murphy and Jones 2016).

Impacts

Defining Impact

In order to assess the impact of fire peer challenge, we developed an impact assessment framework which identified four main components of the peer challenge process: resources, activities, impacts and outcomes (Fig. 5.1).

The resources include those involved in designing and managing the process and promoting the offer to the sector. The members of the team are a vital input into the process, offering a blend of experience and expertise tailored to a service's needs. Finally, fire services themselves invest time and staff resources in producing the OpA, hosting the peer challenge and learning from and responding to the team's recommendations.

Fire peer challenge includes a range of activities such as a set-up meeting and preparation, analysis of documents, onsite activity involving interviews and focus groups with staff, councillors, partners and stakeholders, verbal feedback, and a written report to fire and rescue services.

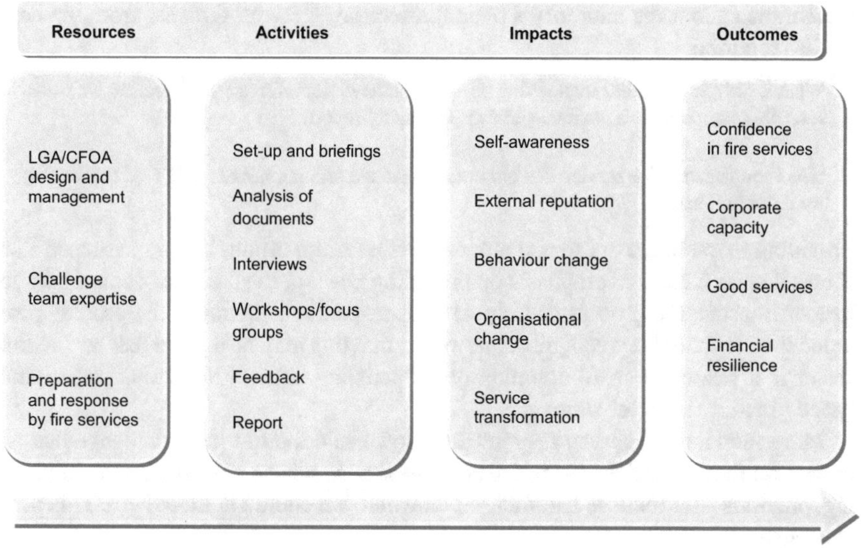

Resources	Activities	Impacts	Outcomes
LGA/CFOA design and management	Set-up and briefings	Self-awareness	Confidence in fire services
	Analysis of documents	External reputation	Corporate capacity
Challenge team expertise	Interviews	Behaviour change	Good services
	Workshops/focus groups	Organisational change	
Preparation and response by fire services	Feedback		Financial resilience
	Report	Service transformation	

Fig. 5.1 Impact assessment framework

Our previous analysis of corporate peer challenge in local government (Downe et al. 2013) suggested that there are five key areas of impacts which are all equally relevant for fire and rescue services.

The process encourages:

- Greater self-awareness
- Improved external reputation
- Behaviour change
- Organisational change
- Service transformation

Given the resources invested and the activities carried out, impacts in these areas should ultimately lead to outcomes. It is difficult to establish a direct causal link between the impacts of fire peer challenge and better outcomes. This is because it often takes time for better outcomes to become apparent and there are so many other factors which influence outcomes beyond the fire peer challenge. It is also difficult to measure an outcome such as increased confidence in the fire service. The rest of this section examines the evidence relating to impacts of fire peer challenge.

Self-Awareness and External Reputation

The most important area of impact was in providing reassurance, in particular to chief fire officers and chairs, that services were on the right track. More than three-quarters (79%) of survey respondents reported that the challenge provided reassurance about the authority's overall direction of travel. Officers from the case studies reported:

> What it did for us: rather than giving us anything new, it reinforced the direction we were travelling in, it's quite a positive and complimentary report.

> It has confirmed to the service that our cultural change programme has delivered the results we thought it had.

Providing reassurance to fire and rescue services is important, but our evidence also shows that an increased emphasis on providing new approaches/ideas could help to further improve the process as only 41% of respondents believed the process provided this. It should be recognised, however, that this may be a 'hard ask' as the fire sector is a relatively small community and existing networking should mean that 'good practice' is widely known.

More than half of survey respondents (56%) said the fire peer challenge had an impact on the service's self-image. For one service whose performance is improving, previous peer reviews had focused on where we could get more help. This peer challenge:

> Focussed on areas where we were creating some ground-breaking work and this has raised the levels of confidence within the service.

Where the report was positive, sharing the key findings with staff and having the chance to celebrate success had helped with morale:

> We took the headlines from the report to all levels of the organisation and you can see the shoulders go back and the head up for all staff, including fire fighters. It has improved morale.

It is difficult to know the impact of a positive report on those beyond the service, but two-thirds of respondents thought that it had improved their service's reputation in the sector.

Behaviour Change

Around a third of survey respondents (34%) thought that the process identified issues that they were aware of but which had been difficult to address without an external stimulus. As a result, the process led to changes in the way that some people worked and operated in the short term which is likely to have medium-longer term benefits.

Nearly half (46%) of respondents reported that the fire peer challenge had positively affected scrutiny by councillors, 37% said it had influenced member–officer relationships and 26% that it had led to changes in approaches to member development.

The case studies showed that councillors found it valuable to have an independent, external view on their service. Officers valued the way in which challenge teams had brought to councillors' attention the fundamental issues facing their services. Examples included the scale of the financial challenge they faced and the need to improve governance arrangements. Officers said that teams had reinforced some of the messages they had been giving councillors and this external validation was a powerful means of highlighting the need for action. According to one officer:

> It was a chance to gather any concerns and ensure that they were all on-board for the change. Are you robust enough? Have you thrashed everything out? It was helpful for an outsider to ask these questions.

In another service, the challenge changed the way in which councillors were engaged in going forward. More priority is now put on getting all councillors engaged in the change process from the earliest stage by improving their understanding of detail and the possible implications.

Organisational Change

Three-quarters of survey respondents reported that the fire peer challenge had led to improvements in the way the service is run, in particular improving the quality of services (cited by 66% of survey respondents) and organisational and workforce development (65%). There was less reported impact on staff engagement (42%) and public engagement (29%).

Interviewees generally reported that the challenge process had more impact on corporate issues than on operational matters. For example, nearly half of survey respondents (46%) believed that the fire peer challenge had an impact on their approach to partnership working. In one service, the peer team highlighted that they had involvement with too many partners and were over-committed. This made the service reflect on how to get more value out of partnerships and to improve the way in which meetings were ran.

Service Transformation

While the majority of impacts were on corporate processes, fire services also received detailed advice on particular parts of the service where they requested support. So, in one service, the team outlined ways in which call handling could be improved. Fire safety was the main area for improvement in another service and the team suggested good practice in other services who were managing their resources in a different way. Finally, another service was advised to re-evaluate the number of home fire safety visits they were doing which was lower than their peer group. Officers appreciated receiving this information on notable practice, so they could follow-up on this after the challenge. Some issues such as making greater use of IT in supporting new ways of working were prevalent across a number of services.

The fire peer challenge does not seem to have had a strong impact on financial areas. Only 25% agreed that it had impacted on financial planning, 17% thought that it had impacted on their use of resources (e.g. buildings, IT, etc.) and just 8% on the service's procurement processes. A third agreed that it had some impact on the way the service responds to the cuts. The most positive result was that 55% agreed that it had a positive impact on their service's efficiency/transformation programmes.

The current pressures on budgets mean that these are challenging times for fire and rescue services. It is important that the OpA and fire peer challenge adds value by enabling services to make maximum use of available resources and to continue to deliver improvements. Therefore, more attention could be paid to the potential for efficiency, innovation and collaborative working. The financial element of the process could be expanded so that peer teams review existing financial data which assess how resilient services are in the current environment.

Conclusions

The OpA and fire peer challenge is viewed by the majority of respondents as working well. The process provides an independent assessment, feedback on how a service can improve and a valuable opportunity for networking with experienced staff and councillors from within the sector. It has delivered external validation that many FRSs have valued and is seen as being credible by the sector, mainly because of the calibre of the teams it attracts.

The results from our survey show that the process is highly valued by the sector with nearly all respondents (96%) agreeing that it helps to maintain the reputation of the sector. Respondents also reported that OpA and fire peer challenge:

- Provides a structured and consistent basis to drive continuous improvement (88% of survey respondents)
- Provides councillors and chief officers with information that allows them to challenge their operational service delivery to ensure it is efficient, effective and robust (88%)
- Is an effective way of ensuring the sector as a whole improves (82%)
- Is a transparent mechanism for providing challenge to fire and rescue services (79%)
- Is a robust mechanism for providing challenge to the sector (71%)

More than three-quarters (79%) reported that the benefits of fire peer challenge outweigh its costs and 56% said that the impact has been more positive than previous inspection regimes. The peer challenge process aims to be about learning and examining how services are delivering for their communities. An important difference is in the approach. Respondents found the peer challenge to be more open and honest than the previous regime which meant that services found it easier to follow up on recommendations.

Seven in ten respondents (71%) thought that the balance between operational issues and corporate leadership/capacity was about right. This means that the process is providing some reassurance at the strategic level, but this isn't replicated at the operational level. The case studies revealed some concerns about picking up operational problems:

> The whole process is more of an organisational assessment than an operational assessment.

> The balance is not right. If there were problems between staff or with members, the peer challenge would probably pick that up. If there was an operational problem, I'm not sure if it would find it.

It would have been the role of the inspectorate to provide input on operational issues and a minority of interviews missed the operational assurance they provided. The majority felt, however, that the re-introduction of an inspectorate would be an unnecessary and retrospective move so long as services were engaging with the OpA and peer challenge process properly. There is a responsibility on fire and rescue services, the CFOA and the LGA to ensure that processes are sufficiently robust and to be aware where risks to performance may be occurring. The peer challenge process could be improved by tailoring it so that, for example, a challenge could focus only upon the operational aspects based on a risk-assessment in one service while a strategic organisational challenge could be undertaken in another service.

The process relies on the integrity of a fire and rescue service to undertake an honest and accurate self-assessment that can be used as a base for the challenge team to investigate critical issues. There is a concern that some services view the process as an opportunity to present strengths while hiding areas of weakness. The challenge team may be able to uncover this but a short visit of four days makes this difficult.

Fire peer challenge is designed to be forward-looking and should therefore provide ideas for improving the delivery of the service. Only half of respondents reported that useful sources of advice and support were given (and only 4% strongly agreed). While it is part of the team's job to highlight examples of notable practice, it is important to get the balance right between seeking out examples of notable practice and sufficiently challenging the service on their operational performance and leadership/corporate capacity.

Once notable practice has been highlighted, much more needs to be done to disseminate these examples across the sector so that all services can share learning on issues which are relevant to them (Murphy and Greenhalgh 2013b). This could lead to additional guidance within the OpA as well as expanding the knowledge base on which challenge teams currently give advice. We heard that team members generally provided examples of good practice from their own organisations only.

As a follow-up visit is not part of the process, it is the responsibility of each service to devise an action plan in response to the report and to implement any changes. There is no external body which checks whether any recommendations are followed up. We feel that in order to 'close the loop', each service should set out how they have responded (or not) to recommendations within the report so that there is transparency on where the process has led to change.

While the process is aimed at improving and not judging a fire and rescue service, a number of interviewees missed having a score or label, which demonstrated how they were performing. This reflects the competitive nature of the sector, the wish to show improvement over time and to compare performance against their peers. We heard that some fire services compare their performance with others within family groups (such as the metropolitan fire authorities), but there seems to be a lack of knowledge about the performance of fire services across the country. Where performance data exist, these should be used to compare how fire authorities are performing across a range of indicators at the local, regional and national level.

This chapter has presented both the strengths and weaknesses of the fire peer challenge approach as perceived by those who have experienced it. We have shown how FRSs have embraced the sector-led approach as a tool to help them improve, but questions remain on whether the process is 'hard hitting' enough and if it can provide sufficient assurance for politicians and the public. As FRSs undertake a fire peer challenge every three years, there is potentially a heightened risk that bad practices may go undetected and/or services may react slower to performance issues, compared to previous regimes. Our evidence suggests that, in a context of austerity, fire peer challenge provides the 'best' option and a more proportionate form of oversight than that provided by an independent inspectorate.

References

Andrews, R. (2010). The impact of modernisation on fire authority performance: An empirical evaluation. *Policy & Politics, 38*(4), 599–617.

Downe, J., Martin, S. J., & Doering, H. (2013). *Supporting councils to succeed: Independent evaluation of the LGA's corporate peer challenge programme*. London: LGA.

Knight, K. (2013). *Facing the future: Findings from the review of efficiencies and operations in fire and rescue authorities in England*. London: HMSO.

Murphy, P., & Greenhalgh, K. (2013a). Performance management in fire and rescue services. *Public Money & Management, 33*(3), 225–232.

Murphy, P., & Greenhalgh, K. (2013b). Support and intervention arrangements. *Fire, 105*, 13–14.

Murphy, P., & Greenhalgh, K. (2014). Peer challenge needs an independent fire inspectorate. *Fire, 110*, 17–19.

Murphy, P., & Jones, M. (2016). Building the next model for intervention and turnaround in poorly performing local authorities in England. *Local Government Studies, 42*(5), 698–716.

Professor James Downe is a Professor in Public Policy and Management and Director of the Centre for Local and Regional Government Research at Cardiff University. His current research interests are in local government performance regimes, political accountability, sector-led improvement, public trust and the ethical behaviour of local politicians. He has more than 15 years' experience of conducting evaluations on various aspects of local government policy and has published widely from these in leading international journals. He served on the UK Government's Expert Panel on Local Governance and currently sits on the Welsh Government's Public Service Scrutiny Reference Group.

Professor Steve Martin is a Professor of Public Policy and Management at Cardiff Business School and the Director of the Public Policy Institute for Wales. Prior to his current role he established and then led the Centre for Local and Regional Government Research at Cardiff University for more than a decade. Steve has conducted a series of long-term evaluations of major public service reforms and served as an expert adviser to a wide range of government agencies in the UK and internationally. He edits the journal Policy & Politics and has written widely on local government policy and public service improvement.

Dr Heike Doering is a lecturer at Cardiff Business School and a member of the Centre for Local and Regional Government Research. Her research interests focus on the professionalisation of public management, institutional change and comparative capitalisms.

Chapter 6
Collaboration in the Emergency Services

Eddie Kane

Introduction

This chapter outlines the findings of an evaluation carried out for the Emergency Services Collaboration Group, a sector-wide multi-agency collaboration (Parry et al. 2015). The evaluation examined the existing landscape of collaboration and suggested ideas and options for future service re-design and rationalisation. In this chapter, the key findings of the evaluation are outlined, the potential impacts of the new service design proposals are highlighted and some of the issues and options for future change are examined, reflecting on what action has taken place post-consultation and the models being developed to deliver and re-design the challenges they present.

Background

The police, fire and rescue and NHS ambulance services play a vital role in serving and protecting communities. The previous coalition government made a clear policy commitment to ensuring that they continue to deliver for the public and emphasised its belief that greater collaboration across all three services is fundamental to this ambition and that it will improve public safety and save taxpayers millions of pounds. To help further this ambition, the *Emergency Services Working Group* was formed in September 2014 with funding from the Home Office, Department of Health and Department of Communities and Local Government. By providing

E. Kane (✉)
Institute of Mental Health, University of Nottingham, Nottingham, UK
e-mail: eddie.kane2@btinternet.com

© Springer International Publishing AG 2018
P. Murphy, K. Greenhalgh (eds.), *Fire and Rescue Services*,
DOI 10.1007/978-3-319-62155-5_6

strategic leadership, coordination and an overview across England and Wales, the group aimed to improve emergency service collaboration.

The Conservative Party's pre-election manifesto was clear that 'we will enable fire and police services to work more closely together and develop the role of our elected and accountable Police and Crime Commissioners' (The Conservative Party 2015). They further stated that they intend to introduce a duty to collaborate on the three emergency services, so that they will be required to consider collaboration with each other wherever it would drive efficiency or effectiveness, to deliver savings and improve services.

The Conservative Party won the General Election in May 2015. The first Queen's Speech of the new parliament on 27 May 2015 included an announcement that 'New legislation will... improve the law on policing and criminal justice' (Cabinet office 2015) and indicated an intention to include enabling legislation to extend the powers of police and crime commissioners in respect of emergency services.

The new Conservative Government issued a consultation paper in September 2015 that set out some options for closer working between emergency services and a series of questions for responses (HM Government 2015).

The prime minister announced in January 2016 that the responsibility for fire and rescue would be transferred from the Department of Communities and Local Government to the Home Office, indicating a structural change designed to enable collaboration between services by bringing together responsibility for fire and police in the same government department. The stated aim was to 'provide the same clear leadership in central Government that our proposals on emergency services collaboration seek to deliver locally' (HM Government 2016, p.4).

In January 2016, the government published its response to the consultation submissions in *'Enabling Closer Working Between the Emergency Services – Summary of consultation responses and next steps'* (HMG 2016).

The parliamentary bill heralded in the Queen's speech, the Policing and Crime Bill, was introduced to the House of Commons on 10 February 2016.

The bill aims to further reform policing and enable important changes to the governance of fire and rescue services. The changes proposed aim to build capability, improve efficiency, increase public confidence and further enhance local accountability.

The main provision for emergency services is to 'place a duty on police, fire and ambulance services to work together and enable police and crime commissioners to take on responsibility for fire and rescue services where a local case is made'. The Act received Royal Assent in January 2017.

This has the potential to empower locally elected police and crime commissioners, where a local case is made to maximise the scope for efficient and effective police and fire services by enabling the creation of a single employer, facilitating the sharing of back-office functions and streamlining management. The intention is that this will give police and crime commissioners the freedom to deliver the best possible services to the public, whilst maintaining the important distinction between operational policing and fire-fighting, with the law preventing a member of a police force from being a fire-fighter remaining in place and no intention to give fire-fighters the power of arrest.

The government also wants to see police and crime commissioners and NHS ambulance trusts working more closely together to ensure the demand that the police and NHS ambulance services place on each other, on a day-to-day basis, is dealt with in the most effective and efficient manner.

The Research Objectives

In November 2014, the Emergency Services Collaboration Working Group, through the Home Office, commissioned research to evaluate existing and emerging emergency services collaboration in order to establish an evidence base for greater cooperation across the emergency services. This research focused on six emergency services collaboration projects across England and Wales, covering efficient services, effective services and emerging best practice.

In evaluating these projects, the research sought to address the following questions:

- To what extent are projects operating as outlined in their project plans and business cases?
- How has collaboration been achieved?
- To what extent do these collaboration projects support wider public service change?
- How do collaboration projects ensure longevity and become sustainable?
- What lessons have been identified? What evidence is there of successful outcomes (including financial) of these projects?
- Which indicators should be used to monitor collaboration activity in the future?
- What evidence is there of wider sharing of the lessons and of them being learnt?

The fieldwork for the research was conducted between December 2014 and February 2015.

The Research Project

In order to contextualise the primary research, secondary analysis of both policy documents and academic literature was undertaken in the form of a Rapid Evidence Assessment (REA). The following provides a summary of the findings from both.

Findings of the REA

Policy Documents

According to much of the policy literature, resilience, efficiency and reducing bureaucracy are key principles that have underpinned collaboration. Since the introduction of austerity measures for public services, thinking around co-operation between emergency services has intensified. As stated by the Emergency Services Working Group, 'with an increasing demand for some of our services, coupled with the current and expected restrictions on funding, collaboration provides opportunities to truly innovate and save money', what was once considered exceptional performance required in the event of a major incident is now becoming part of the expected response to budget cuts. The Knight Report (2013), whilst placing most of its emphasis on the need for rationalisation of structures within the fire service, acknowledged that 'national level changes to enable greater collaboration with other blue-light services, including through shared governance, co-working and co-location, would unlock further savings'.

In more recent documents, collaboration has also been viewed not just as potentially realising savings but also as a duty and obligation. This was evident in policy and legislation across all the blue-light services going back to a statutory responsibility to collaborate and achieve interoperability enshrined in the Civil Contingencies Act 2004 reinforced by the expectation of the current Policing and Crime Bill.

Similar or enhanced duties are placed on the services at a national level. The exercise of these duties is supported by the former National Policing Improvement Agency (NPIA) guidance on Multi-Agency Interoperability of 2009, and again in the Joint Emergency Services Interoperability Programme's (JESIP) Joint Doctrine Interoperability Framework of 2013, and realised strategically through the work of the local resilience forums.

There are common areas identified as being suitable for collaboration. The Department of Communications and Local Government report *Future Control Room Services Scheme: National picture of fire and rescue authority improvement plans* (DCLG 2014) acknowledges that there are gains to be made by sharing control rooms. An earlier publication from the Local Government Group Going the Extra Mile (March 2011) offers a review of efficiency models within fire and rescue services, ranging from the fairly obvious, such as shared procurement, to the highly innovative, including a new Directorate in Cornwall County Council which brings together the Fire and Rescue Service, the Crime and Disorder Reduction Team, Environmental Health, Licensing, Port Health, Coroner's Services and Trading Standards.

Amongst the complexities identified for services in achieving effective collaboration is the multifaceted line of responsibility locally and nationally. This has particularly been the case for police and fire authorities. However, there is also a suggestion that these barriers can be overcome. Her Majesty's Inspectorate of Constabulary (HMIC) suggests that there are some good examples of collaborative working between the police with various external bodies (including the private sector) where a shared vision, strong leadership and a sense of compromise can help to manage the impact of differing structures (HMIC 2012). In both fire and ambulance reports, the key focus has been on co-responding. In 2008, the Department for Communities and Local Government reported that there were 99 co-responding stations in 18 fire and rescue services in England but that it varied across Fire and Rescue Authorities (FRAs) and was concentrated across a few counties (DCLG 2008).

Collaboration has been reported to be fragmented and slow to progress. For example, HMIC has expressed concern about the ad hoc way collaboration is being implemented noting that 'forces are developing a clearer picture of how they intend to collaborate, and with whom: but the anticipated savings, level of ambition and approach vary considerably across England and Wales' (HMIC 2012, p.9). Justification for this has often been the incompatibility of organisational structures and culture. However, whilst recognised in various reports, these barriers are not seen as insurmountable.

There has been some financial support to strengthen emergency services collaboration. This is evidenced by government funding, for example, the DCLG Transformation Challenge Fund and Fire and Rescue Transformation Fund which invested £30 million in resources and £45 million in capital in 2015–2016 to assist in the development of collaborative projects. Similarly, the Police Innovation Fund has awarded £9.2 million to 12 projects in 10 force areas.

Academic Literature

Most of the academic literature tends to focus on major incidents, small case studies or responding to major incidents. Relevant findings in academic literature support the concerns found in policy reports. In particular, the differences related to organisational culture found between communities of practice can create numerous barriers to effective co-working – though these can be expected to decrease as practical exposure to different communities becomes the norm. The problem of organisational culture seems to be universal. Research from New South Wales (Australia) identified similar barriers to effective collaboration, reflecting the findings of the policy literature (DCLG 2008). Importantly, although there were perceived improvements in joined-up working, a number of hurdles remained. These included the perennial concerns of competing organisational requirements, concerns regarding resources and professional identity. This research suggests that it is important to build inter-organisational trust, rather than organising funding and management in a way that fuels competition, and underlines the value of treating people with fairness and respect as a good way of achieving stakeholder support for operational change.

These cultural differences spill over into the use of technology so that even when IT or communications systems are re-designed to remove communication and data-sharing barriers, such problems can persist. Sanders found that 'The varying social world ideologies within emergency response... have influenced access to emergency technologies and their stored information and in turn, have created an ideological disconnect between how these technologies were designed to function, and their in-situ application' (Sanders 2014, p.472). Emergency interoperability, therefore, is as much a social process as a technological one.

Where researchers consider initiatives to enhance collaboration within a single service, cultural differences would be expected to play a smaller role and can certainly be overcome. In relation to innovation in three police force areas, Allen and Karanasios (2011) highlight that this process can be managed carefully with a staged approach to change. They emphasise that barriers to innovation can be replicated across forces. In addition, they state that learning and sharing lessons about how collaboration is achieved is critical to success. As to how far the experience of working together in the event of civil contingencies can facilitate a more general move towards day-to-day collaboration, research suggests that there is a contribution to be made if it is handled with due concern for organisational differences. Rogers (2011) argues that, 'sharing of best practice is of vital importance, even more so amongst organizations that have been historically entrenched in the specific needs of service delivery for local areas with distinct needs, and have perhaps even been forced into institutional cultures of competition for resources in what has until the last decade been underfunded, but is now laden with intrusive efforts to reform'.

Evaluation Methodology

Collaborative projects can be complex to evaluate. To ensure that the evaluation was comprehensive, a mixed-method approach was applied to effectively assess existing and developing emergency service collaborations. The approach combined qualitative and quantitative data collection from primary and secondary sources. This included interviews, focus groups, surveys and reviews of performance reports, academic literature and policy documents. The practical possibilities of mixing inquiry methodologies contributed to, and reflected, the complexity and diversity of the challenges involved in inter- and intra-service collaboration.

Case Study Selection

The case study areas were selected from a list of national projects contained within an overview of collaboration produced by the Emergency Services Collaboration Working Group and agreed with that group. The following criteria were used to determine the sample:

- Covered all three areas of project focus – efficient services, effective services and emerging best practice

- Had a geographical coverage encompassing rural and urban areas – national areas
- Had projects within single local authorities and projects across local authorities

All three emergency services were covered – ambulance, fire and police – as well as local authority partners.

Interviews with Emergency Services Staff

Fifty-one in-depth, semi-structured interviews (face-to-face and telephone) were held with senior staff responsible for developing, managing and monitoring emergency services collaboration projects across the six areas. These include Chief Fire Officers, Chief Constables, Police and Crime Commissioners (PCC), Chief Executives of Ambulance Trusts, Local Authority Chief Executives and elected members.

The interview topics covered:

- Motivation behind collaboration
- Features of collaboration projects
- Impact on service delivery
- Barriers/enablers
- Measuring success
- Lessons learnt
- Sustainability

Focus Groups

To explore more general issues around emergency services collaboration and to capture the views of operational staff, three focus groups were held in Manchester, Lincolnshire and Surrey/Sussex. The focus group themes were designed to further develop the interview themes from a front-line/operational perspective.

Economic Impact

An economic evaluation was undertaken, based on data from the six case study areas. The purpose of conducting data analysis and economic evaluation was to (i) systematically understand financial and outcome data in the selected case study areas, (ii) analyse the business cases in terms of clarity in presenting costs and benefits that can be independently verified, (iii) develop outcome measures that can be used to measure success or otherwise of the projects, (iv) recommend a uniform way of presenting business cases and indicators of success and (v) encourage the areas to quantify the wider social benefits of their projects.

Surveys

We also carried out two surveys:

- Survey of representative bodies: In order to broaden the research, a short online survey of representative bodies was conducted. This covered those trade unions and professional organisations that represented employees of one or more of the emergency services and local authorities.
- Public perception: Given that the remit of all three services (and local authorities) is to serve the public, a short survey was undertaken to determine their opinions of collaboration. A survey of 1069 individuals was conducted to gather the public's ideas on the subject. The survey topics included awareness of, confidence in and importance of emergency services collaboration.

Key Findings

The evaluation led us to some overarching conclusions:

- Collaboration is driven by both efficiency and effectiveness and by the need to save money.
- Effectiveness is not just related to achieving savings – it is also about delivering better services and outcomes for the public.
- Collaboration has been achieved in a number of ways and with a range of participants. There is no 'one model' – it works on an area-by-area basis that reflects local need.

Collaboration across England and Wales is 'patchy' due to a number of factors that include:

- The nature and timing of funding streams that do not always allow all services the opportunity to collaborate at the same time or to the same degree
- Local 'politics' that can inhibit or stimulate collaboration – this includes trade unions
- Inconsistent messages across government departments
- Legacy issues from previous collaborations that can impact on the appetite for further collaboration

A number of common lessons have been identified in the six case study areas and are included in Table 6.1:

Table 6.1 Lessons from the case studies

Where emergency services collaboration is successful, it is grounded in a clear, shared vision between partners.
Local political (non-partisan) endorsement is critical in providing support.
It is often key individuals driving collaboration and this requires that appropriate communications and transfer of responsibilities are in place when those personnel move on.
Appropriate, universally agreed governance structures are essential in the management and development of collaboration.
In collaboration between services (inter), it is important that due consideration is given to collaboration within the same service (intra).
In aligning services through collaboration, retaining 'brand' identity is both a common aspiration and a key challenge.
There is positive public backing for collaboration but a lack of public awareness about what currently happens.
Sustainability of collaboration is linked to local decisions around future direction (e.g. underpinning what exists or expanding reach).
Collaboration would be given further momentum if linked to key performance indicators. These could cover things such as response times, public confidence, capital expenditure, crime and detections rates, cost savings, etc.
Future funding is key to sustainability and expansion – a range of options exist, for example, more funding from central government, commissioning of services and franchising of existing models.
Early outcomes appear favourable (e.g. response times in Lincolnshire and Manchester), but it is too early to measure impact with any degree of certainty.
Data is patchy, inconsistent and not linked to targets.
Evidence of successful financial outcomes within the project areas is limited and will take time to be realised; therefore, it is difficult to provide a conclusive economic analysis.

Collaboration projects also support wider public service change and links in to local and regional developments in other areas, for example, social care.

In addition, there were a series of graded recommendations. The recommendations cover suggestions for greater collaboration (supported to varying degrees by research participants) as well as suggestions for promoting enablers and removing barriers. These were broken down into five types:

• Increasing collaboration
• Removing barriers
• Promoting enablers
• Improving data quality
• Improving business planning

We then split them into three levels, characterised by:

• Evidence of breadth and level of support
• Ease (or difficulty) with which recommendations can be implemented from a practical point of view
• Degree of effort, will and compromise required by strategic leaders and/or central government in order to bring about further collaboration

The three levels are summarised as follows:

Level 1

- Characterised by substantial support and deliverability
- Underpinned by both primary and secondary data
- Issues that are fairly straightforward to address
- Tasks that can be achieved with moderate effort/will by those partners who have an appetite/need for collaboration or further collaboration

Level 2

- Characterised by strong support
- Underpinned by both primary and secondary data
- More complex issues to manage/overcome
- Issues that require a degree of negotiation and compromise in order to achieve

Level 3

- Characterised by mixed support
- Key barriers to manage/overcome
- Ambitious and sweeping change
- Decisions that will require addressing at a senior level in order to embed collaboration consistently (at all levels) across England and Wales

Current Developments

Since the publication of the Crime and Policing Bill and *Enabling Closer Working Between the Emergency Services* (HM Government 2016) in the first half of 2016, there have been elections for police and crime commissioners in 41 of the 43 territorial forces in England and Wales (May 2016). These elections appear to have prompted an initial flurry of activity to explore the business case for using the potential new powers in the Crime and Policing Bill to develop new governance and delivery structures for emergency services. Notably, a number of territories have commissioned consultants to offer support in exploring the options, benefits and challenges the alternatives offer.

To date, a good deal of what is emerging covers old and relatively safe ground. For example:

- Merger of support services and some operational areas including estates, fleet, procurement, payroll and pensions, information sharing and operational (prevention and response)
- Strategic targets for Police Transformation Fund Bids, for example, IT and Control Rooms
- Other areas include training, communications and media, finance and legal services, human resources and corporate performance

There is an informally reported, wider recognition that there are clear opportunities to be gained from co-location as well as standardising and aligning processes in support services. The current operational prizes being identified are mainly at a tactical level – greater appetite for prevention activities over more response-related activities. The benefits of better information sharing are becoming more widely acknowledged with opportunities existing at a number of levels; some involve IT solutions but most are about trust and leadership and local existing working practices.

The more complex area and the one that new legislation aims to enable progress in is overall governance.

Three broad options are being explored by those organisations that have publically commissioned work:

- Option 1: PCCs take over governance of their local Fire and Rescue Authority and two employers maintained the 'Governance' model.

     The benefits of this model are seen as:

Economic:

- – Potential savings in relation to Secretariat costs resulting from FRA being abolished
- – Potential acceleration of opportunities to share procurement, estate and other assets could reduce costs

Efficiency and Effectiveness and Public Safety:

- – More direct accountability to the public which could increase public confidence and visibility
- – Reduction of the cost and improved effectiveness of public consultations linked to the Fire and Rescue Act 2004
- – Single-governance structure could speed up decision-making and accelerate collaboration opportunities that could improve efficiency and effectiveness, especially relating to back-office support services where a lead employer model could be adopted
- – Could remove barriers to data and information sharing for prevention and protection activity
- – Single-governance structure could lead to a more integrated service, leading to better value for money and more outcomes

The risks generally identified include:

Economic:

- – Potential transition costs, including costs of new support services currently provided in kind by local authority

Efficiency and effectiveness and public safety:

- Potential risk that policing issues will dominate the new arrangements and fire-related decisions will not get priority
- Association with the police could damage trust in fire-fighters (there is some supporting evidence for this from the USA, for example Wilson and Grammich 2015)
- Need to adjust scrutiny mechanisms to account for new responsibilities could take time
- Potentially strong resistance from fire unions which could lead to industrial action and delay operational collaboration
- Levers for more radical collaboration may still be constrained given the absence of a single-employer model or significantly more integrated operational structures
- Fire may weaken links to local government, the NHS and other organisations which enable services to make a wider social contribution

- Option 2: PCCs take over governance of their local Fire and Rescue Authority, and a single employer created the 'Single Employer model.
  The benefits of this model are seen as:

Economic:

- The ability to streamline upper tiers of management

Efficiency and effectiveness and public safety:

- Remove the barriers that can prevent the full potential of fire and police collaboration, including the need to draw up contracts and collaboration agreements to share back-office services
- Potential ability to deploy operational resource and budget more effectively
- Potential ability to revisit and harmonise terms and conditions that will enable more flexibility and new delivery models over time, such as the ability to have single terms for community-focused roles
- Improved ability to allocate funding for joint prevention and response initiatives, greater links between crime pattern analysis and strategic fire assessments

The risks generally identified include:

Economic:

- Likely to have transition costs to move to a new model and potentially the most complex of the new models to implement

Efficiency and effectiveness and public safety:

- Complexity of managing a single-employer model operating under distinct statutory and non-statutory arrangements for police and fire relating to terms and conditions, pay and dispute resolution may lead to a reduction in additional benefits from this model relative to other options
- Likely to be highly controversial and result in industrial action that could delay collaboration

- How misconduct and professional standards matters will be dealt with, as police and fire currently have different requirements and standards

- Option 3: PCCs are represented on the Fire and Rescue Authorities – the 'Representation' model.
  The benefits of this model are seen as:

Economic:

- Quick and low cost to achieve

Efficiency and effectiveness and public safety:

- Less contentious
- Can enhance collaboration opportunities if there is a good working relationship and shared vision between police and fire
- Full voting rights ensure they can take part in discussions and decisions in a meaningful and effective way
- Will foster closer relations between police and fire

The risks of this model are generally seen as:

Economic:

- PCC representation across FRA sub-committees could impose significant burdens on PCC and Office of the Police and Crime Commissioner and duplicate cost and activity, increasing overall governance costs.

Efficiency and effectiveness and public safety:

- Still requires formal collaboration agreements and decision-making could be too slow
- Depending upon the arrangements, if the PCC is in fundamental disagreement with the other fire authority members, there could be an impasse or the PCC could be overruled
- May confuse lines of accountability and performance management

These options in many ways mirror some of the key features of the consolidation models underpinning the relatively large scale of mergers in emergency services in the USA in recent years. Wilson and Grammich (2015) recently characterised these levels as:

Nominal Consolidation

Nominally consolidated departments usually do not have integrated police and fire services nor do they have cross-trained public-safety personnel. These departments typically have a public-safety director overseeing separate police and fire divisions within a single department. They may maintain shared facilities, training, or dispatch resources between police and fire divisions (p. 363).

Partial Consolidation

Involves a limited integration of police and fire services. Partially consolidated departments have a limited number of cross-trained public-safety officers who are trained to perform both police and fire duties. Such personnel work alongside separate police and fire personnel in the same department (p. 363).

Full Consolidation

Involves a complete integration of police and fire services. Fully consolidated departments .... These agencies consolidate the management and command of both police and fire services into a single entity (p. 363).

Discussion

One of the most striking findings in the evaluation carried out for the Emergency Services Collaboration Group came from the survey of over a 1000 members of the public. They strongly supported closer working between emergency services, and even more strikingly, they actually believed it was already happening to a far greater degree than is in fact the case. The combination of public expectation with the potential of new enabling legislation augurs well for the development of new models of integration and delivery for emergency services. However, it is worth reflecting on the lessons from the USA where mergers of emergency services, particularly fire and police, have been commonplace in recent years. The Wilson and Grammich study reported that *'in recent years, a growing number of communities have consolidated their police and fire agencies into a single "public-service" agency. Consolidation has appealed to communities seeking to achieve efficiency and cost-effectiveness'* (2015, p. 361). However, they also found that *'Some communities have even begun to abandon the model. Exploring the reasons for disbanding can help cities considering the public-safety model determine whether it is right for them'* (2015, p. 361).

If consolidation of fire and police and indeed other emergency services, under whatever local model is chosen, is to be effective in England and Wales, the lessons learnt elsewhere need to be used to help test the robustness of new planned arrangements. Lessons learnt from the collaboration arrangements already in place in England and Wales can also help shape future new initiatives. However, as the Research into Emergency Services Collaboration (England and Wales) Report (Parry et al. 2015) highlights, the current collaborations fall some way short of the ambition underpinning the government's intention to drive a radical delivery and economic set of benefits in this area. It will be interesting to analyse the early alternative models that are produced for local consultation. It will be especially interesting to examine the extent to which some of the fundamental issues that led to the reversal of consolidation in the USA and elsewhere have been addressed or ignored.

The future operation of integrated emergency services depends on a rigorous and honest assessment of the challenges, a clear plan owned by all stakeholders and most importantly a clear rationale for the integration that must stretch well beyond financial drivers and must not sweep the very real barriers to success under the table.

References

Allen, D., & Karanasios, S. (2011). Critical Factors and Patterns in the Innovation Process. *Policing (Oxford): A Journal of Policy and Practice, 5*(1), 87–97.

Cabinet Office and HM Queen. (2015). *Her Majesty's most gracious speech to both houses of Parliament at the state opening of Parliament 2015*. London: Cabinet Office.

Department for Communities and Local Government. (2008). *Current practice and prospects for FRS co-responding: Fire research series 14/2008*. London: DCLG.

Department for Communities and Local Government. (2014). *Future control room services scheme: National picture of fire and rescue authority improvement plans – October 2014 update*. London: DCLG.

Her Majesty's Inspector of Constabulary. (2012). *Increasing efficiency in the police service: The role of collaboration*. London: HMIC.

HM Government. (2015). *Enabling closer working between the emergency services – consultation document*. London: HM Government.

HM Government. (2016). *Enabling closer working between the emergency services – summary of consultation responses and next steps*. London: HM Government.

Home Office. (2016). *Policing and crime bill*. London: Home Office.

Knight, K. (2013). *Facing the future: Findings from the review of efficiencies and operations in fire and rescue authorities in England*. London: Department for Communities and Local Government.

Parry, J., Kane, E., Martin, D., & Bandyopadhyay, S. (2015). *Research into emergency services collaboration*. Sheffield: Emergency Service Working Group Research Report.

Rogers, P. (2011). Resilience and civil contingencies: Tensions in northeast and northwest UK (2000–2008). *Journal of Policing, Intelligence and Counter Terrorism, 6*(2), 91–107.

Sanders, C. B. (2014). Need to know vs. need to share: Information technology and the intersecting work of police, fire and paramedics. *Information, Communication & Society, 17*(4), 463–475.

The Conservative Party. (2015). *Strong leadership, a clear economic plan, a brighter, more secure future: Conservative party Manifesto*. London: Conservative Party.

Wilson, J. M., & Grammich, C. A. (2015). Deconsolidation of public-safety agencies providing police and fire services. *International Criminal Justice Review, 25*(4), 361–378.

Professor Eddie Kane is Director of the Centre for Health and Justice at the Institute of Mental Health, University of Nottingham. He currently leads teams delivering major national and international research programmes including HEFCE Catalyst and College of Policing, large grant-funding programmes covering the development of evidence-based interventions at the health-justice interface and policy review programmes in forensic services. He is currently funded by the British Foreign Office and Chinese Government to develop new training approaches for mental health workers including the translation and validation of both Chinese and English language education materials. He continues to advise Government on aspects of Home Affairs and High Risk Offenders. He led the University of Nottingham team that developed the National Knowledge and Understanding Framework for personality disorders.

He was previously the Department of Health's principal adviser on personality disorder (PD) services where he led the development of the national PD strategy including the Capabilities Framework Workforce and training development plan. He was the National Director of High Security Psychiatric Services. He also worked as the Director of NHS Performance and Mental Health for London and as Director of Mental Health for the Northwest and West Midlands regions of England. He has been an NHS Trust CEO and held board-level positions in a variety of public, private and voluntary organisations.

Chapter 7
Governance and Accountability to Service Users

Julian Clarke

Introduction

The relationship of fire and rescue services (FRSs) with stakeholder groups has become increasingly important as public services have 'modernised'. This chapter will specifically examine the governance and local accountability arrangements of FRSs in the UK. It will focus on the way in which FRSs are accountable to the populations for which they provide services. It will examine also how these roles and relationships have evolved and the changing governance and accountability arrangements that have guided and enabled the scrutiny of fire services in the modern era.

As public protection, risk prevention, risk mitigation and the desire to change public behaviour has increasingly become a feature of their work, services have been required to engage with the public much more closely and regularly. In an era of declining resources, instant mass communication, 24 h news and the burgeoning influence of social media, FRSs have been required to adapt the way they relate to their public and local communities. The changing nature of these roles and the increased challenge of reputation management within an era of absolute and relative decline of resources available for the service will be illustrated with reference to various attempts by FRSs to both engage more closely with their public and to broaden the range of services and activities they offer to that public.

This chapter will examine the relationship of fire and rescue services with their service users. It will also indicate how the relationship between central and local authority and the different kinds of accountability involved in these relationships constrains representative local democracy, and it examines critically commissioning and delivery of services and future public involvement in planning and shaping the services provided.

J. Clarke (✉)
Edgehill Business School, Edgehill University, Lancashire, UK
e-mail: clarkej@edgehill.ac.uk

© Springer International Publishing AG 2018
P. Murphy, K. Greenhalgh (eds.), *Fire and Rescue Services*,
DOI 10.1007/978-3-319-62155-5_7

One of the central problems that will be discussed is the divide between expert allocation of scarce resources and a range of localised 'community' interests which may or may not be consistent with each other, raising the question common to all democratic politics: what kind of accountability? This question is examined in the second part of this chapter where different accountability mechanisms are discussed. The first part of the chapter first looks at a range of conceptual considerations that provide a context for discussing FRS accountability. The 2012 National Framework in which accountability to local populations emerged as a fully formed but vaguely defined duty for FRS is examined. Part 1 then tracks back to find the source of this duty and briefly looks at the emergence of accountability as a central feature of local governance.

Part 1: Accountability – Scepticism and Policy Development

Five Decades of Scepticism

The concept of accountability for FRS no longer simply refers to formal budgetary competence and financial probity, but it has become bound to both management accountability and performance measurement and to the notions of engagement, consultation and participation (Kloot 2009). Bovens (2010) usefully distinguishes between accountability conceptualised on the one hand as a good thing that everyone favours and which, may involve many different activities but is vaguely defined in terms of its outcomes. On the other accountability can be defined as the existence and operation of specific mechanisms, protocols and sanctions. But the problems only start here. Defining what is effective or 'real' accountability in Bovens' second sense is highly contentious and deeply politicised.

From Arnstein (1969) through writers such as Cockburn (1977) and Craig and Mayo (1995) to Mowbray (2011), the notions of public service engagement and accountability have been subject to critical and sceptical examination. The basic question is: to what extent and at what level can individuals, groups of individuals and local interest groups shape or alter policy decisions and changes in actual service delivery and to what extent should they be able to do so? Should both the employment and service delivery patterns of a fire and rescue service be solely determined by the expert knowledge of a cadre of senior managers moderated (perhaps) by experienced but non-expert elected members? Or should more participatory or deliberative forms of democracy (Mutz 2006) or perhaps a greater emphasis on co-production determine the distribution of services and the employment of staff (Boyle and Harris 2009)? These questions become even more important during a period of declining resource.

Arnstein's famous ladder (1969) describes a continuum that ascends from the placation and/or manipulation of a population through to its participatory empowerment. At the bottom of the ladder, consultation and engagement are designed to defuse discontent and opposition and manage expectations. At the top of the ladder, decisions are taken directly by an informed and active community. While it is relatively easy to define the kind of consultation, which is done merely to placate, it is less easy to provide a useful model for participatory empowerment as opposed to representative democratic decision-making. The Arnstein continuum has been slightly updated by Svara and Denhardt (2010) to include such concepts as co-production, but these modifications do not solve the accountability problem. But as Denhardt and Denhardt say in the latest edition of their landmark book *The New Public Service: Serving not Steering*:

> public servants, are called upon to be responsive to all competing norms, values and preferences or our complex governance system. Accountability is not and cannot be made simple. (Denhardt and Denhardt 2015: p143)

Scepticism about large organisations consulting and engaging with service recipients and being accountable is a good thing. Cynicism or the denial that any form of consultation or engagement is worthwhile and that there is no such thing as 'real' accountability is probably not.

Consultation, Engagement and Involvement: Principals and Agents

In discussions of consultation, there seems to be agreement that engagement and involvement should be a broad process that includes a variety of types of contact and information provision. Consultation, however, is usually a formal process that deals with specific sets of issues (Sheedy 2008). A general definition of engagement leaves open a series of questions about who does the engaging and with whom.

Involvement and participation were watchwords under recent New Labour Governments with the public service organisations seen as the instigators of engagement processes with 'the community' or communities, whose nature and variety was often ill-defined (Clarke and Kaleem 2010). Beyond a certain point, consultation and engagement presuppose an active, well-informed citizenry capable of professional levels of service monitoring and analysis. Participative or deliberative democracy requires such a citizenry and a completely different set of decision-making processes. Accountability conceived within a framework defined in this way would require a forum or mechanism with real powers, which might conflict with the formal mechanisms of representative accountability (fire authorities) that are relatively speaking indirect. As we will see in Part 2, service users usually seek direct accountability when existing services are going to be changed and/or appear to be threatened. Continuous engagement is rare except amongst a minority of citizens.

In public administration theory, accountability can be conceived in terms of the principal/agent problem. Principal–agent theory (PAT) defines a problem for all public service organisations. How does the principal, the service user, the public or electorate make sure that their objectives are realised (assuming of course that there is a well-defined collective interest)? The assumption is that there is no necessary alignment between the interests of public service managers and those of the principals. The principal–agent argument hinges on the nature of the incentives that principals can deploy to make objectives align. This in turn becomes a problem of the control and distribution of information relevant to decision-making (Laffont and Martimort 2003). Although developed to analyse the economic behaviour of different categories of individuals mainly in private for-profit organisations, principal–agent theory can be read through into the analysis of public sector, not-for-profit organisations. Miller, for example, argues that:

> Principal agency theory has allowed political scientists new insights into the role of information asymmetry and incentives in political relationships. It has given us a way to think formally about power as the modification of incentives to induce actions in the interests of the principal. (Miller 2005: p203)

This insight is important when considering the governance of UK FRS where there is usually an elected fire authority composed of (perhaps knowledgeable and well-informed) amateurs, which is collectively the principal and a highly skilled, professional fire and rescue service management team, which is the agent. Looked at from another perspective, local tax payers and electors are the principal(s) and the fire authority and service are the agents.[1] This raises a question about how a fire authority represents individually or collectively the interests or needs of the population served by their FRS. How does the principal (citizens/voters) ensure that the agent (elected councillors on the fire authority) do what they want them to do? Or how does the fire authority (in this second case the principal) get the FRS senior managers (the agent) to do what it wants? Examination of the two instances confirm the argument that the principal–agent theory: 'is in fact a highly flexible family of models rather than an overarching set of assumptions and results' (Gailmard 2012: p1). These questions will be addressed in more detail in Part 2.

The 2012 National Framework and Good Governance

A new National Framework for UK Fire Services in England[2] was published in 2012. The development of the Framework began in 2010 with the production of a series of Fire Futures papers including one that specifically pulled together one aspect of the coalition government's localism focus with ideas about accountability, greater transparency and the development of a monitoring competence.

> The Service must…meet the evolving risks to communities and the changing needs of citizens. This cannot be done without bringing decision making and accountability much closer to citizens and communities. (DCLG Fire Futures 2010: p3)

Although there is reference to governance in the Framework document, there is no elaboration of the idea. Thinking about governance in relation to fire and rescue services has come from a different source. Good governance as envisaged by, for example, the CIPFA/SOLACE framework (2001) incorporates developments in thinking and practice around a much wider range of accountability 'competences' than envisaged by traditional public administration: a model defining a linear relationship between the elected members of local and national bodies and the paid public servants who deliver services with an electoral feedback loop from service user voters to the elected members (Hood 1991, also Lynn 2001).

The CIPFA guidance has developed since it was first issued in 2001 and both constitutes and embodies an important part of the development of the concept and practice of public service governance in the UK. The 2004 Governance Standard emphasises the relationship between elected representatives, FRS management and community groups:

> Their responsibility [the management and elected membership] is to ensure that they address the purpose and objectives of these organisations and that they work in the public interest. They have to bring about positive outcomes for the people who use the services, as well as providing good value for the taxpayers who fund these services. They have to balance the public interest with their accountability to government and an increasingly complex regulatory environment, and motivate front-line staff by making sure that good executive leadership is in place. (CIPFA ODPM 2004 Standard)

The CIPFA/SOLACE guidance (2007) has been incorporated, at least nominally, into local service delivery thinking and practice by organisations as diverse as Birmingham City Council (2014) and the Peak District National Park Authority (2012). It has also been adopted widely by Fire and Rescue Authorities, which have produced codes of corporate governance consistent with the framework (see, e.g. Derbyshire Fire Authority (2014), Surrey FRS (2013) and Cheshire FRS (2012)).

The conception of good governance outlined depends on who gets to define public interest, value for money and positive outcomes for service users. The CIPFA framework does not answer this question.

Development of National Regulation and Accountability

The election of 'New Labour' in 1997 saw a major series of transformations in public service regulatory regimes. These can be conceptualised for the purposes of this chapter as the requirement by various services to develop and demonstrate a series of accountability competences some of which were familiar and some not. Broadly, they can be characterised in the following way for fire and rescue services:

- Management/planning competence
- Financial competence
- Risk analysis competence
- Service delivery competence
- Resilience and continuity competence
- Community safety/prevention competence
- Human resource competence
- Community engagement and accountability competence
- Equality and diversity competence

This chapter is concerned only with community engagement and accountability.

The idea of (direct) accountability to service users emerged slowly within a range of regulated competences after the local government modernisation process began in the late 1990s. The development and maintenance of these competences are not necessarily consistent with each other and may pull fire authorities and fire services in different directions. Potential conflicts have become a more pressing problem as real resources are reduced and services have to be reworked. The major legislative changes underpinning the development of regulation have been detailed earlier. The Local Government Act 1999 and the Fire and Rescue Services Act 2004 have a limited amount to say about engagement and accountability. But the former does lay down a duty to consult with community representatives with respect to the delivery of Best Value.

Two important regulatory regimes emerged during the Labour administrations of 2001–2010. The Comprehensive Performance Assessment (CPA) and the Comprehensive Area Assessment (CAA) were corporate performance management schemes that dealt with a number of traditional competences such as budgetary and operational competence. They also elaborated the accountability of FRS to the central government modernisation project and contained a drive towards community partnerships and accountability. The white paper *Strong and Prosperous Communities* (DCLG 2006) indicated that local people would have:

> …more say in running local services by reforming the best value regime to ensure that local authorities and other best value authorities inform, consult, involve and devolve to local citizens and communities, where appropriate. (DCLG 2006, p26)

The white paper was followed by the Local Government and Involvement in Public Health Act 2007, which was unclear about the extent of required consultation (by whom and about what). This was clarified by Statutory Guidance. *Creating Strong, Safe and Prosperous Communities* (DCLG 2008a) laid out in some detail 'a duty to involve'. It was accompanied by *Citizens in control* (DCLG 2008b), which was supposed to be the ordinary person's guide to making local decision-making accountable. The *Duty to Involve* followed in 2009.

Within 2 years, all this was gone, revoked by the incoming coalition government that left just the basic *Best Value Duty* (to consult) in place but removed everything else. It might be asserted that the idea of the Big Society and the Localism Act 2011 provided a replacement that did more to empower citizens at a local level. The relationship between the Localism Act and the Fire Futures conclusions about the need for accountability, however, is ambiguous because the former did not contribute specifically to a discourse of public sector accountability. On the one hand, it gave local groups the right to challenge for the provision of some aspects of service delivery (and encouraged potential for-profit private providers) and also gave fire services more freedom to extend the range of services they provided through a 'general power of competence' (DCLG 2011).

FRS Policy Development and Regulation

The regulatory regime that applied to FRS developed out of the Bain/Lyons/Young review report (Bain 2002), which discussed accountability and consultation very much in terms of inter-organisational relationships. Engagement with service users is discussed at some length (Bain 2002) but in the context of public education about risk and partnership rather than accountability to those service users.

The 2004 Fire Services Act that followed the review required that fire and rescue services produce Integrated Risk Management Plans (IRMPs). The first local-level stakeholder consultations were held in 2003/2004 (ODPM 2004). The 2004 National Fire Services Framework trailed the requirement of fire services to participate in the Comprehensive Performance Assessment and also assigned responsibilities in relation to floods, decontamination, and search and rescue (ODPM 2004). There is no mention of accountability in the Framework and consultation is again mainly discussed in terms of a relationship between formally constituted national and local bodies.

Comprehensive Performance Assessment reports very rarely referred to accountability. The majority, however, commented favourably on the adequacy of individual fire authority and service engagement with the public and the detail of their consultation policies, plans and practices. But at least one report does ask a key question: how has consultation shaped the priorities of the service? (Audit Commission 2008). This question was raised again in the organisational reports for FRS conducted under the Comprehensive Area Assessment regime.

Accountability might have appeared centre stage in the transition from CPA to Comprehensive Area Assessment in 2009. But FRSs were to be assessed in relation to:

> ...the priorities and objectives set out in the Fire and Rescue Service National Framework, assessing the extent to which individual fire and rescue services are delivering against the framework, effectively balancing their prevention, protection and response functions. This will include considering how well equality and diversity are fully integrated into all aspects of the service. The Audit Commission will also assess the impact and effectiveness of the service's contribution to broader partnership outcomes in the LAA. (Audit Commission 2009, p.33)

Although engagement and consultation are referred to in the organisational reports, there was an incomplete translation of the more general policy aims relating to involvement and accountability outlined above into the actual assessments. For example, FRSs were included in Local Area Agreements but in a limited way (Matheson et al. 2011). There is commentary on engagement and consultation and a question about whether concerns expressed at engagement events or from consultations feed into service change. But there is very little about accountability.

By contrast, the 2012 National Framework contains two whole sections on assurance and accountability to communities. The Framework covers three principal areas: safer communities, accountability to communities and assurance. The key terms in the section on accountability are engagement, transparency and scrutiny,

particularly in relation to the IRMP. The community should have sufficient information to be able to challenge the decisions constitutive of the IRMP through the fire
authority, which in turn should be open to public scrutiny (DCLG 2012, p16).

The post-2010 era is supposedly one of 'light touch' regulation where there is
limited independent assessment. Both CPA and CAA are long gone and have been
replaced by self-assessed Assurance Statements prepared by individual FRSs. These
follow the guidelines set out in the 2012 Framework and claim to make FRS
accountable to the populations that they serve (see, e.g. assurance statements from
Manchester FRS (2013) and Cheshire FRS (2013)).

The assurance statements produced in 2013 by FRSs are fairly brief documents
that summarise how each FRS is responding to the criteria laid out in 2012
Framework.

They, however, reference ancillary documents that indicate how fire authorities
and fire services have approached the policies and practices explored in this chapter.
On the whole, these sets of documents demonstrate that the authorities and services
have quite thoroughly internalised and embedded modes of assessment that were
externally imposed during previous phases of regulation. In particular, the assurance statements clearly document engagement and consultation strategies.

Only a focussed and determined member of the public, however, is likely to track
down and digest the full implications of these reports. The issues of transparency
and accessibility become even more important when changes to service configuration are considered during the IRMP planning process as will be seen in Part 2 of
this chapter.

Part 2: Local Accountability

Accountable to Whom and in What Way?

The ideas and policies described in Part 1 have helped to shape what can be called
current FRS 'accountability practices'. We need to assess how these individually
and severally make an FRS accountable to it service users and partners. Each practice area will be examined briefly to see how they contribute to Bovens' two ideas
of accountability; principally his second notion, which is accountability to a forum
with the potential for sanctions. A central question is: in what way do the accountability practices of a fire authority and an FRS produce an Integrated Risk
Management Plan that meets the fire and rescue needs of the population served by
an FRS and is seen to do so by that population?

Fire authorities are the principal forum (and probably the only one in Bovens'
second sense) in which FRSs make themselves accountable to their service users.
But this accountability is representative and therefore indirect. Accountability is
also sought through formal consultation, various kinds of direct public engagement
and involvement, and in some cases, empowerment strategies although empowerment
strategies do not seem to have been renewed since 2010 (Cheshire FRS 2009).

Accountability to partner organisations takes a variety of forms. Partners are included in consultation and engagement but also relate to FRS through partnership governance structures. We also have to take account of the way in which FRSs respond to public protest of various kinds; how this links to the other accountability practices. Response to protest is examined in the context of local objections to specific local allocations of resource.

Fire Authorities

Current FRS governance arrangements were established by the Fire and Rescue Services Act 2004, which set out the conditions for the formation of fire authorities within the existing local government framework. Broad duties for dealing with fires and road traffic accidents and promoting fire safety were laid out. Additional emergency duties outside the fire and road remits were also included (c21 part 2). In England, fire authorities are the only legally constituted local-level accountability forum for FRSs. It is important to ask if fire authorities are fulfilling duties as they might be defined by the discussion undertaken in Part 1. Have they, for example, been able to promote accountability *to communities for the service they provide* (DCLG 2011)?

The important question, however, is whether in what way and to what degree fire authorities can and do hold FRS to account. Fire authorities are made up of elected councillors, who are drawn from constituent local authorities and represent local government wards.[3] They are usually members of one of the main political parties and are themselves potential 'consumers' of fire and rescue services. They also undergo elected member training to support the development of relevant expertise and so are inducted into an existing model of fire and rescue service administration (West Midlands FRA 2013). They are also constrained to operate within the fire and rescue service framework set out by national government.

FRSs have training and member development programmes. The principal aim of these is to ensure that fire authority members understand what is their statutory role and to provide enough information to allow them to understand what decisions are involved in running a fire and rescue service because they have ultimate responsibility for those decisions. Training is usually undertaken by a democratic services department or its equivalent (see, e.g. Manchester FRS 2014). In the Manchester case, one of the competences that fire authority members should develop is to: 'To represent the communities the Authority serves in relation to fire and rescue matters' (Manchester FRS 2014). The term communities seems to be used here, as often in public sector discourse, not to refer to specific and differentiated communities but some public interest, which is differentiated in ways that are left vague.

It is clear, however, from the content of this particular policy document and the associated training regime that the purpose of member development is to make fire authority members competent to understand and discuss the business of the FRS and to take a policy and scrutiny lead. The question here is: to what degree does this induction process institutionalise fire authority members? That is: induct them into a preexisting mindset about the way a fire service should operate and does this affect the way in which members individually and/or collectively represent the communities they were elected to serve?

One of the (perhaps the principal) jobs of the fire authority is to scrutinise and agree a draft of the Integrated Risk Management Plan prior to it being publicised and consulted on. The IRMP is the outcome of risk analysis and the basis for the distribution of resources, and the fire authority has primary formal accountability for the allocations contained in it.[4]

Consulting, Engaging, Involving and Informing

FRSs do not solely interact with their service users via the fire authority. They try to maintain the confidence of potential service users through formal consultation, engagement exercises and the provision of both printed and online information. It is also arguable that the vastly increased fire prevention and home safety work undertaken by all FRSs over the past 15 years is direct public engagement, which did not take place in the same way when FRSs were fire brigades, and the focus was on the protection of property. Home safety assessments have played a major role in the FRSs' modernisation process.

Cheshire FRS, for example, started off simply fitting smoke alarms, but the process developed into a much more comprehensive assessment that was based on a household risk assessment (one size does not fit all) and agency appropriate referrals particularly for older people (Arch and Thurston 2012) and latterly for migrant groups (Clarke 2016). Home safety assessments have been central to FRS engagement strategies and to the development of a range of partnerships.

The perceptions of service users are important. In the first place, most service users only want to be actual users of FRS prevention services in order to have free smoke detectors installed, but service users also want to know that their FRS is competent at the level of risk analysis, planning and prevention. Operational competence has also to be demonstrated. People expect the FRS to get to fires quickly, put them out and if possible prevent injury and death and damage. In the example to be outlined in the next section of this chapter, it will be seen that there is a complex relation between these two areas. These perceptions are complicated by the fact that:

> Many people remain unaware that the FRS is the primary rescue agency in the context of the terrorist threat and also climate change. In a sense, we have become a de facto civil emergency service responsible for fires, transport incidents, crashes, chemical incidents, floods and so on. (McGuirk 2010, p.1)[5]

The situation has been further complicated by funding reductions since 2010. The 2011 Financial Settlement signalled real continuous reductions in FRS funding over the course of the 2010–2015 government. More reductions were indicated following the 2015 election.

The coalition government's deficit reduction and public sector cuts programme has inevitably had consequences for FRS. The *Local savings review guide* (Audit Commission 2010) identified a number of areas where 'efficiencies' could be made. Given that, at the time of the review, staff costs took an average of 75% of FRS budgets (Audit Commission 2010), the review focussed on this area and examined the possibility of reducing the number of staff and reworking crewing arrangements with the possibility of attendant reduction in the number of fire stations and appliances.

Most FRSs have engaged in extensive consultation to seek the views of service users about proposed service changes. Specifically, consultations have focussed on the revision and renewal of Integrated Risk Management Plans. Effective consultation serves not only to test service user, staff and partner views of proposed changes but also to demonstrate that FRSs seek to be accountable.

> With this increased visibility comes an increasing level of public expectation about the quality of service we provide and how we meet the needs of the diverse range of communities we serve….Public understanding, involvement and support will be particularly important in the coming years as challenging decisions need to be made about the future of the Service at a time of considerable pressure on finances. (Cheshire FRS 2012, p.2)

Many FRSs have detailed strategies that lay out how consultation and engagement will be undertaken (see, e.g. Manchester FRS 2012). Easy access to information such as web pages, newsletters and draft planning documents is emphasised. Accredited consultation via online questionnaires and panel meetings provides a summary of public responses that have a statistically valid basis (Cheshire FRS 2012). Formal consultation processes have sought to undertake several related but different tasks: first, to assess the degree of confidence in and satisfaction of service users with FRS, second to assess response to changes such as charges for smoke alarms and third to seek the views of service users about specific changes in local allocation of resources such as fire station closures or changes in crewing patterns and cover patterns (see, e.g. Cheshire FRS 2014). Arnstein's ladder of participation is mentioned in more than one strategy document (Manchester FRS 2012, Cheshire FRS 2012)!

All FRSs work within a range of partnerships, both long term and fixed duration. Partnership accountability is complex because the FRSs have commitments to both delivery partners and service users. Partnerships have been one of the areas of work that have extended the FRS role beyond firefighting and rescue work, and they have been important in developing preventative safety and more broad-based community strategies.

Youth engagement has been a major theme across all FRSs. Current fire cadet schemes date back to the mid-1980s, and all FRSs have these (Fire services youth training organization 2016) (http://www.fsyta.org.uk/about-us/). Involvement with the Prince's Trust has led to FRS delivering 20% of the Trust youth programmes. Youth engagement is seen to be:

> One of the most effective ways of achieving a safer community is to work with young people from groups at particular risk of becoming involved in crime and disorder, arson and deliberate fire-setting. This in turn helps those young people who are at risk through unhealthy, chaotic and potentially harmful lifestyles, to get into work, training or education. (www.princes-trust.org.uk)

Accountability to partners has been developed through a mix of mechanisms. Where the partnership has a statutory footing such as the Local Resilience Forums, FRS partners develop plans and capabilities according to a set risk indicators coordinated by the local authorities (see, e.g. Cheshire Resilience Forum 2014). Other formal partnerships tend to be with other public sector bodies and the voluntary sector. Local older people's charities and the voluntary sector domestic violence organisations are examples of cooperation where mutual accountability is achieved through partnership boards (see Clarke 2016 for more detail on the range and governance of FRS partnerships).

The Integrated Risk Management Plan and Different Perceptions of Risk

The advent of austerity in 2010 has made it necessary to take policy and planning decisions that alter local distribution of FRS resources. All FRSs have been legally obliged to produce risk management plans that detail this kind of change at regular intervals since 2004. The 2012 National Framework requires that FRS:

> identify and assess the full range of foreseeable fire and rescue related risks their areas face, make provision for prevention and protection activities and respond to incidents appropriately.

and do this within a context where they:

> work in partnership with their communities and a wide range of partners locally and nationally to deliver their service [and]...[are] accountable to communities for the service they provide. (DCLG 2012, p.7)

Risk analysis has a number of aspects: the development of an overall set of fire risk assessments for the area served, which is followed by the differential allocation of resources to different parts of that area in terms of fire cover (fire stations, appliances, different crewing arrangements). Prevention work that has been universal may now be targeted through risk analysis and connected to advice to households and businesses on how to manage their own risk. Enforcement work also involves risk analysis. It is the first of these – differential allocation of resources – across the area of operation, which is of principal interest here because it raises key accountability issues. In an era of expenditure cuts where there may be quite dramatic differential assessment outcomes, the issue of resource allocation may become more problematic and locally politicised.

Reductions in funding have coincided with and can be rationalised by a country-wide decline in the number of fire injuries and fire deaths (Knight 2013). But as changes have been proposed over the past 5 years or so, the effect of reductions on fire service response times have become a matter of debate.

The FRS view of risk and how it is to be handled is contained within the IRMP and associated documentation. How to respond to is risk determined by available resource and judgements about differential levels of risk as they are distributed across the area of operation. The risk management models in use will take a range of factors into account. The Cheshire FRS Community Risk Management Model, for example, takes into account at least 10 sets of factors, which have to be weighed in risk assessment (Cheshire FRS 2016). Drafts of the IRMP produced by the senior management team have to be approved by the fire authority and are often the subject of vigorous debate.[6] A fire authority as a collectivity has to recognise the constraints under which IRMPs are now produced and individual members find it difficult to engage in special pleading in response to protest from specific community groups. Fire authority members also have to recognise limitations in their ability to criticise certain technical aspects of the risk assessment process and also the problems of arguing the case for specific interest groups.

After 2010, there were many local protests about resource reallocation. Why should such protests arise? Protests about austerity-induced changes have focussed on closing of fire stations, reduction in the number or relocation of fire appliances and changes in crewing arrangements.[7] Ultimately, however, risk is seen from the users' point of view in terms of increased response times: how long does it take a fire appliance to get to a fire? Longer response times are seen to be the effect of some or all of the changes just mentioned.

This concern is reflected in the consultation results reported by various FRSs. How widely this concern is felt by most citizens is unclear. Some of the detailed responses to be found in consultation reports indicate a degree of knowledge that is not common amongst average service users and may relate to professional exper- tise. Where response time has been a concern, the rationale is straightforward: the longer it takes a fire appliance to get to a fire, the greater the risk is of fire damage, fire injury or fire death.

In at least one case, a website with an online forum was developed. The website argued that changes to crewing the local fire station implied that:

> Along with job losses this means when a fire occurs these people will have to leave their place of work, travel to the fire station and get changed into their protective clothing before they can attend to the fire, making call-out times significantly longer.

and

> ...With every minute counting in a serious fire these cutbacks are putting people's lives in danger and we believe might lead to the complete closure of the fire station in the future if suitable part time staff can't be found. (Save Knutsford Fire Station 2014)

The website was accompanied by a petition and a letter sent to local decision- makers which objected to the 'downgrading' of the fire station from full-time to on-call crewing. The Cheshire FRS chief fire officer attended a Town Council Meeting within 2 weeks of the website appearing and explained why the decision to change the crewing of the station had been made. He denied that there was any intention to close the station. No change was made to the crewing decision.

Research carried out by the DCLG, which shows that between 1996 and 2006 aver- age dwelling fire response times worsened from five and a half to six and a half min- utes (DCLG 2009) and by 2014/15 had declined by more than a further minute (DCLG 2015). The Entec report for the Home Office (1999) indicates a negligible increase in likelihood of fire death between a 5- and 10-min response time. Calculations, however, made in a subsequent report indicate that the increase might have resulted in five additional deaths per year in the 1996–2006 period; although during this time, there was actually a fall in fire deaths of 142 per year (DCLG 2009).

Explaining the increase in response times has proved difficult:

> [in 2009] increasing traffic levels were found to be a major factor behind increasing response times. Traffic levels have decreased since 2008, yet response times continued to increase until 2010–11, albeit increasing more slowly, indicating that there must have been other factors behind the increases in average response times until 2010–11.

A range of other factors were proposed in 2009 – increased emphasis on firefighter safety, more careful driving and call handlers asking for more information than formerly. None of these seem to explain the increase satisfactorily (DCLG 2009, pp.46–47).

The Fire Brigades Union (FBU) believed that it had a clear explanation. The modernisation programme that followed the 2004 Act and the replacement of the 1985 National Fire Standards by Integrated Risk Management Planning have been at the root of the problem. Quick response has been replaced by an emphasis on safety and prevention and cutting the number of firefighters. Response standards are set locally and are uneven across the country. The fundamental argument is that response time matters and that increases lead to more death, injuries and fire damage (Fire Brigades Union 2010). This view is supported by the DCLG work (DCLG 2009:82). The FBU report does not mention the overall decrease in fire deaths, which can be shown to be related to safety and prevention work (Arch and Thurston 2012). Currently, the Cheshire and other FRSs have risk-assessed response time targets of 10 min.

Protest, Perception of Risk and Subsidiarity

There are two main perceptions of risk at work (a third if we count in the FBU view as defining risk differently). The first is the FRS conception embedded in risk management planning for the FRS operational area. It is based in differential risk assessments for different parts of the area. Allocation of resources is based on these assessments and response time targeted on this basis. Service user risk assessment, as based in recent protests, is different. Service users see increased response times as increased risk and, if changes are made at the level of an individual fire station, as specifically an increased risk to the people served by that fire station. The two conceptions of risk are not compatible. Unless service users can show that resource allocations are in error from the point of view of an overall FRS risk analysis, it is difficult to see why an FRS should change them.

Direct local accountability at fire station level could probably only work with a volunteer service financed out of (very) local taxation supplemented by borrowing or grants. There are FRSs in the USA that fit this model (see Firehouse 2016). Implementing anything like this in the UK is extremely unlikely for a range of politico-legal reasons. There are volunteer fire stations in the UK, but these are part of the officially designated FRS (Daily Mail 2012) and are resourced and governed by a fire authority.

The concept of subsidiarity is important: taking specific policy and service delivery at the lowest appropriate level and, in each specific case, working out how those decisions can be arrived at. Despite the attempts of recent Labour Governments to encourage involvement and latterly the coalition to define and encourage localism, the public services are mainly organised and delivered by large organisations that remain primarily accountable to the state (the current government).

In the case of fire authorities, service delivery is hedged around with legal considerations principally laid out in the FRS Act 2004, which strictly limits the devolution of substantial lower-level decision-making by the local fire authority. It is also dependent on levels of finance provided by central government. In any case, the principle of subsidiarity does not usually define what kind of specific structures of accountability will be established; these are imposed by the state and often give little room for manoeuvre.

Police and Crime Commissioners

The replacement of fire authorities by elected police commissioners may change the way in which representative democratic institutions work and, in particular, respond to popular protest. But elected commissioners whose primary role is to govern local police services are unlikely to change the way in which FRSs carry out risk assessments or allocate resources. Whether they will be able or even try to integrate FRSs and police engagement activities is a completely open question.[8]

Conclusion

The first part of this chapter dealt with the context in which current FRS accountability practices have developed since the turn of the century. It started with critical views that have been expressed about the possibility of 'real accountability' to service users. Since the late 1960s, a range of writers have been sceptical about public sector accountability. These writers have seen consultation as a largely empty or manipulative process. This chapter argues that while a critical and sceptical stance is a good thing, cynicism and the assertion that there is no such thing as 'real accountability' is probably not. The concept of accountability is not straightforward, and its translation into policy and then into action brings many difficulties. Mark Bovens' dual conception of accountability is useful because it avoids some of the argument about what is 'real accountability'. That debate, however, does not simply disappear, but it currently hinges around what kind of accountability representative democracy provides. There are extensive arguments about the desirability and possibility of participatory local democratic control within a representative system. But their application to the way in which an FRS would be accountable to the population it serves is unexplored.

The principal/agent problem indicates how complex accountability is. When discussing local accountability, the key elements are access to information and an engaged citizenry that is able to use that information. The complexities of the current situation can be characterised in terms of several different principal/agent relationships:

- First between service users and their fire authority and FRS senior management
- Second between a fire authority and the senior FRS management
- Third between central government, fire authorities and FRS senior management

Each of these relationships has different content, different information flows and different accountability structures. The focus of this chapter has been on the first relationship as mediated by the second. But we have recognised that the overall shape of these relations is partly defined and certainly constrained by the third.

The 2012 National FRS Framework defined accountability to services users as a central aspect of good FRS governance. But neither the Framework nor the CIPFA guidance on accountability that many public sector bodies have incorporated into their governance documentation provides much information about what might count as accountability in terms of public interest, value for money and positive outcomes for service users.

Policy defining how FRS should engage with and become accountable to their service users emerged quite slowly during the period of comprehensive public sector regulation and inspection between 1999 and 2010. Legislative support for local accountability through engagement and involvement did not arrive until 2008–2009. The regulatory regime driven by successive Labour Governments disappeared after the 2010 election to be replaced by a 'light touch' regime. The Cameron-inspired Big Society initiative led nowhere. But the assurance statements required of FRS after 2010 do follow the guidelines set out in the 2012 National Framework and claim to make FRS accountable to the populations that they serve.

Part 2 examines how FRS local accountability practices have emerged. Again if we adopt Bovens' two-part definition of accountability, then only those FRSs that are answerable to a fire authority or an equivalent local authority committee meet his second criterion, accountability to a forum. Consulting, engaging and involving in a range of other ways are important in informing service users and getting feedback from them, but in terms of representative democracy they are ancillary activities.

The main question asked is to what degree fire authorities can and do hold FRS to account on behalf of service users? Examination of the documentation guiding training regimes indicates that the purpose of member development is to make fire authority members competent to understand and discuss the business of the FRS and to take a policy and scrutiny lead. It is important to ask if training and development induct them into a preexisting mindset about the way a fire service should operate. It is not clear what the balance of influence is between fulfilling their legally defined role and taking on board, for example, the outputs from consultation and engagement and from direct public protest.

Fire authorities and FRS do try to maintain the confidence of potential service users through formal consultation, engagement exercises and the provision of both printed and online information. The change of emphasis from property protection to prevention and human safety has been key. The specific fire safety and in some cases more general home safety work undertaken by all FRSs over the past 15 years is direct public engagement, which did not take place in the same way when FRSs were fire brigades, and the focus was on the protection of property.

Fire authority accountability to local populations has been constrained by a variety of conditions. At a national level, these are existing law and regulation and finance, currently austerity and budget reductions. Changes to law and the regulatory regime in the first decade of the century brought about profound changes in the way that FRSs operate. FRSs and their fire authorities were accountable across a wide range of operational areas to national government via inspections and subsequent reports. Since 2010, regulation has become more 'light touch'. Currently, the main constraints are financial and relate to the production of assurance statements. These do contain duties of accountability to 'communities', but these duties are expressed in a very general way, and it is not clear what test of adequacy might be applied.[9]

Since 2004, each FRS has been required to produce and renew a dedicated Integrated Risk Management Plan. With budgetary reductions signalled from 2010 onwards, all FRSs have had to rework resource allocations, which has meant fire station closures, changes in the number and distribution of appliances and changing in crewing arrangements. Local protest has been generated around these changes with a principal focus on increased FRS response times. There has been a measured increase in FRS response time since the late 1990s, which it is estimated may have led to a small increase in death, injury and damage. But at the same time fire deaths have actually decreased by a substantial number, driven mainly by prevention work.

Expert assessment of risk is founded on different assumptions than those of individual service users and specific communities. FRSs are accountable for their overall assessment of risk in their area of operation. It is difficult to see how an FRS can be accountable to specific communities or interest groups for failing to make changes to proposals that have attracted objections unless it can be shown that overall risk management planning is in some way faulty. Subsidiarity in the sense of devolving fire service provision to local communities is not possible within the current national legal framework. It is not easy to see how it might work (other than in very isolated and/or very sparsely populated areas) although there are examples in the USA of very small local fire services.

Changes in the configuration and governance of the emergency services may change the nature of fire and rescue accountability, as has happened in Scotland, but until such changes are proposed or happen in England their effects cannot be assessed.

Notes

1. The principal–agent distinction in the case of UK fire and rescue services is complex because national governments produced a series of regulatory regimes in the first decade of the century; it can be argued that national government ministry is the key principal and each fire authority and its associated service are the

agents. There is also a strongly unionised cadre of front-line firefighters that has sought to maintain its own employment conditions during a period of organisational change and financial austerity, which also might be considered as an agent.

2. By 2012 following devolution, Scotland and Wales had joined Northern Ireland in having their own frameworks and/or strategies. The fourth national framework applies to England only.

3. The exception to this are counties where there is no separate fire authority, and the county council itself constitutes the fire authority and delegates most functions to the chief fire officer while retaining overall responsibility. There are also slightly different arrangements in London.

4. Fire authority members are likely to be influenced by the outputs from consultation and engagement and to direct public protest, but it is beyond the scope of this chapter to determine how this varies from member to member or authority to authority. It might constitute the basis for future research.

5. Steve McGuirk was until 2015 Greater Manchester's County Fire Officer (Chief Fire Officer).

6. This comment is supported by observation over the period of a year at one of the fire authority's meetings. Other fire authorities may be different, and there may be no sustained debate, but anecdotal evidence from colleagues involved in similar research suggests not.

7. An Internet trawl revealed more than 30 protests recorded in local newspapers and on local news programmes. The Knutsford protest described below is typical.

8. There is considerable ongoing debate about the potential changing nature of these accountability and operational arrangements but that lies outside the scope of this chapter.

9. At the time of writing, both a team from the Home Office and a team of academics are reviewing the nature, contents and purpose of the statements of assurance.

References

Audit Commission. (2010). *Local savings review guide*. London: Audit Commission.

Arch, B., & Thurston, M. (2012). An assessment of the impact of home safety assessments on fires and fire-related injuries: A case study of Cheshire Fire and Rescue. *Journal of Public Health, 35*(2), 200–205.

Arnstein, S. (1969). A ladder of citizen participation. *Journal of the American Planning Association, 35*(4), 216–224.

Audit Commission. (2008). *Corporate assessment Cleveland Fire Authority*. London: Audit Commission.

Audit Commission. (2009). *Comprehensive area assessment framework document*. London: Audit Commission.

Bain, G., (2002). *The future of the fire service; reducing risks saving lives: The independent review of the fire service*. Norwich: TSO.

Bovens, M. (2010). Two concepts of accountability: Accountability as a virtue and as a mechanism. *West European Politics, 33*(5), 946–967.

Boyle, M., & Harris, D. (2009). *The challenge of co-production: How equal partnerships between professionals and the public are crucial to improving public services.* London: National Endowment for Science, Technology and the Arts (Great Britain).

Birmingham City Council. (2014). *Local code of governance.* Available at http://www.birmingham.gov.uk/governance.

Cheshire FRS. (2009). *Community empowerment strategy.* Winsford: Cheshire FRS.

Cheshire FRS. (2013). *Statement of assurance 2012–13.* Winsford: Cheshire FRS.

Cheshire FRS. (2014). *Making Cheshire safer: Integrated risk management plan for 2014/1.* Winsford: Cheshire FRS.

Cheshire FRS. (2012). *Consultation and engagement strategy.* Winsford: Cheshire FRS.

Cheshire FRS. (2015). *Member training and development programme 2015/2016.* Winsford: Cheshire FRS.

Cheshire FRS. (2016). *Making Cheshire safer.* Winsford: Cheshire FRS.

Cheshire Resilience Forum. (2014). *Emergency response manual.* Winsford: Cheshire FRS.

CIPFA/SOLACE Working Group. (2001). *Corporate governance in local government - a keystone for community governance.* London: CIPFA.

CIPFA/SOLACE. (2007). *Delivering good governance in local government framework.* London: CIPFA.

Clarke, J. (2016). Beyond authority: Public value, innovation and entrepreneurship in a UK fire and rescue service. In J. Liddle (Ed.), *New perspectives on research, policy & practice in public entrepreneurship* (Vol. 6). Bingley: Emerald.

Clarke, J., & Kaleem, N. (2010). Equality, vulnerability, risk, and service delivery: equality improvement in fire and rescue services. *International Fire Service Journal of Leadership and Management, 4*(2), 12–22.

Cockburn, C. (1977). The local state: Management of cities and people. *Race & Class, 18*, 363–376.

Craig, G., & Mayo, M. (1995). *Community empowerment: A reader in participation and development.* London: Zed books.

DCLG. (2006). *Strong and Prosperous Communities.* London: TSO.

DCLG. (2009). *Review of fire and rescue service response times.* London: TSO.

DCLG. (2008a). *Creating strong, safe and prosperous communities.* London: TSO.

DCLG. (2008b). *Citizens in control: Fire futures localism and accountability report.* London: TSO.

DCLG. (2010). *Fire Futures.* London: TSO.

DCLG. (2011). *Accountability and transparency for fire and rescue authorities.* London: TSO.

DCLG. (2012). *Fire and rescue national framework for England.* London: TSO.

DCLG. (2015). *Fire incidents response times: April 2014 to March 2015, England.* London: TSO.

Daily Mail. (2012). No need for a fireman's pole! World's tiniest fire station is just big enough to store a single emergency LAND ROVER, 13 January, London.

Derbyshire Fire Authority. (2014). *Corporate code of governance.* Littleover: Derbyshire FRA.

Denhardt, J., & Denhardt, R. (2015). The New Public Service revisited. *Public Administration Review, 75*(5), 664–672.

Fire Services Youth Training Organization. (2016). See http://www.fsyta.org.uk/about-us/.

Fire Brigades Union. (2010). *It's about time, why emergency response times matter to firefighters and the public.* Kingston-upon-Thames: FBU.

Firehouse. (2016). *What is The Smallest Fire Dept. That You've Seen?* http://www.firehouse.com/forums/t71117/.

Gailmard, S. (2012). *Accountability and principal-agent models, Oxford handbook of public accountability.* Oxford: OUP.

Home Office. (1999). *Response time fatality rate relationships for dwelling fires (Entec UK Limited).* London: TSO.

Hood, C. (1991). A public management for all seasons? *Public Administration, 69*(1), 3–19.

Kloot, L. (2009). Performance measurement and accountability in an Australian fire service. *International Journal of Public Sector Management, 22*(2), 128–145.

Knight, K. (2013). *Facing the future: Findings from the review of efficiencies and operations in fire and rescue authorities in England.* London: TSO.

Lynn, L. E. (2001). The myth of the bureaucratic paradigm: what traditional public administration really stood for. *Public Administration Review, 61*(2), 144–160.

Laffont, J.-J., & Martimort, D. (2003). *The theory of incentives:The principal-agent model.* Princeton: Princeton University Press.

Manchester FRS. (2012). *Consultation and engagement strategy 2012–2015.* Manchester: Manchester FRS.

Manchester FRS. (2013). *Statement of assurance 2012–2013.* Manchester: Manchester FRS.

Manchester FRS. (2014). *Member training and development policy.* Manchester: Manchester FRS.

Matheson, K., Manning, R., & Williams, S. (2011). From brigade to service: an examination of the role of fire and rescue services in modern local government. *Local Government Studies, 37*(4), 451–465.

McGuirk, S. (2010). From cure to prevention - transformational change in the Fire and Rescue Service. *International Journal of Leadership in Public Services, 6*(4), 18–21.

Miller, G. (2005). The political evolution of principal-agent models. *Annual Review of Political Science, 8*, 203–225.

Mowbray, M. (2011). What became of the local state? Neo-liberalism, community development and local government. *Community Development Journal, 46*, 132–153.

Mutz, D. C. (2006). *Hearing the other side: Deliberative versus participatory democracy.* New York: Cambridge University Press.

Office of the Deputy Prime Minister. (2004). *The 2004/2004 fire and rescue service national framework.* London: TSO.

OPM & CIPFA. (2004). *The good governance standard for public services.* London: CIPFA.

Peak District National Park Authority. (2012). *Code of corporate governance.* Bakewell: PDNPA.

Sheedy, A. (2008). *Handbook on citizen engagement: Beyond consultation.* Ottawa: Canadian Research Policy Networks.

Svara, J., & Denhardt, J. (2010). *The connected community: Local governments as partners in citizen engagement and community building. White paper.* Arizona: Arizona State University.

Save Knutsford Fire Station. (2014). See https://www.change.org/p/george-osborne-mp-save-knutsford-fire-station.

Surrey FRS. (2013). *Governance Review.* Guildford, Surrey FRS.

West Midlands Fire Authority. (2013). *A strategy for supporting and developing members.* Birmingham: WMFA.

Dr. Julian Clarke has a social sciences background including a PhD in social anthropology. Teaching and research originally focussed on ethnicity, race, migration and equality policy. This eventually led to work with the Commission for Racial Equality and the Local Government Association. He was a member of a team that developed the Equality Standard for Local Government and a subsequent assessment programme. A number of FRS took up the Equality Standard and were assessed against the framework. A research interest in FRS management grew out of this work focussed primarily on public service partnership and the creation of public value.

Chapter 8
The Making of a Hero: An Exploration of Heroism in Disasters and Implications for the Emergency Services

Anne Eyre

Introduction

Show me a hero and I'll write you a tragedy. *(F. Scott Fitzgerald)*

References to heroes and heroic acts in disasters are common, particularly when it comes to mass fatality incidents. Accounts and analyses of heroic acts appear in sources as wide ranging as the news media and popular culture through to academic papers and health and safety guidance literature. But although these various sources may be using the same term, are they all talking about the same kinds of behaviour and attributes?[1]

This chapter begins by examining the psychological and social context of major emergencies as potentially traumatic events and the significance of this for understanding disaster-related actions and behaviour. In some cases, reactions to disasters may be as much about spontaneous, instinctive human responses as they are about the measured implementation of pre-prepared emergency procedures. It is important to acknowledge this if we are to understand, anticipate and interpret extraordinary and heroic acts where people risk their own lives in responding to the needs of others.

The newsworthiness and other social and political agendas served by the discourse of disaster heroes will be briefly referred to along with the wider consequences of being labelled a hero. For a member of the public who becomes the

---

[1] In this chapter, the terms 'major emergency' and 'disaster' are used interchangeably to refer to large-scale incidents placing life and/or property in danger, often involving multiple casualties and/or fatalities and likely requiring multi-agency response and assistance.

An earlier version of this paper was published in the International Fire Service Journal of Leadership and Management, Volume 8, p7–16 (ISSN 1554-3439). We are grateful for permission to include it in this volume.

A. Eyre (✉)
Trauma Training Ltd, Warwickshire, UK
e-mail: anne.eyre@traumatraining.com

© Springer International Publishing AG 2018
P. Murphy, K. Greenhalgh (eds.), *Fire and Rescue Services*,
DOI 10.1007/978-3-319-62155-5_8

victim-cum-hero, finding oneself unwittingly caught up in a life-threatening event can be life changing enough, but in the aftermath, there may be additional costs associated with identifications of heroism such as additional survivor guilt.

Members of the emergency services may be described as everyday (albeit often reluctant) heroes to the extent that they deliberately enter environments of risk as part of their ordinary duties, but their actions in the context of major emergencies may attract additional attention and analysis in the following days and weeks. This chapter considers the renewed focus on risk, health and safety within emergency response, prompted by a series of major incidents and investigations within the UK, and the consequences these have had for revisiting the interpretation and guidance around acts considered heroic within the law, custom and practice.

Understanding Disaster Experiences and Heroism

Exceptional events often generate exceptional individual and social reactions. To understand disaster-related behaviour, it is important to appreciate how such circumstances can impact on the perceptions, experiences and social responses of those involved in them and what this means for questions of heroism. Focussing on disasters as psychological and social experiences gives some insight into understanding when behaviour is truly heroic and its implications.

Major emergencies or disasters are, thankfully, relatively abnormal events rather than everyday occurrences within communities. Psychologists and sociologists highlight how behavioural responses reflect the ways in which they differ from normal, everyday experiences and routine emergency response. Major emergencies are to a lesser or greater extent:

- Of a different order in terms of emergency procedures and scale of response: the declaration of an event as a major incident or disaster usually triggers a specific set of procedural responses, namely the implementation of 'special arrangements' such as major incident plans. Actions described as heroic tend to fall outside of or beyond prescribed emergency procedures; they are usually spontaneous and unplanned, may be often committed by ordinary bystanders who are not following formal emergency procedures, or they may be committed by emergency responders breaking with or exceeding formal protocols.
- Often described as 'surreal' and quite different in feel from scenes displayed in disaster films or other imaginary scenarios. Many emergency responders reflecting on their first-hand experience of real disaster have emphasised the contrast with drills or exercises, and the impact of such experiences on them both during the event and afterwards. Typical of this is the comment made by a firefighter who responded to the Ladbroke Grove train crash in London, 1999, in which 31 people were killed. Commenting on the initial reactions of shock while gathering up the personal belongings of those who had so suddenly died, the firefighter commented on the feeling of being unprepared for such an encounter: 'In training,

you are shown photos of other major incidents so you are prepared in that way, but nothing in my training prepared me for it when I saw it in real life' (BBC News 1999).

- Experienced as chaotic by those caught up in them and first on scene, at least in the initial phases at the point where sense is being made of what is occurring and before a coordinated emergency response kicks in. Initial emergency calls during the London Bombings, July 2005, typified this reality with first responders facing 'considerable difficulties in assimilating information that is coming in as clearly a very confused incident presented itself' (Hugo Keith QC, speaking at the Inquest, 11 October 2010 (Her Majesty's [HM] Coroner, 2010). In such circumstances, heroic acts may be associated with their bringing leadership or order to bear, or restoring control in the midst of chaos and destruction. The individuals who formed a 'human bridge' to lead fellow passengers to safety in the midst of ferry disasters have been described as 'heroes' in this sense (TNT Magazine 2012; Kent Online 2012).
- Prolonged events, where notions of heroism are associated with notions of endurance as well as spectacular single acts (Smith 2011). The 'Fukushima 50' in Japan has been described in heroic terms. Heroism here has been linked to their continuing work to restore control over the ongoing threats and hazards caused by the nuclear disaster in Japan in March 2011 as well as their initial, self-sacrificing responses at the nuclear plant as the disaster unfolded (Yokota and Yamada 2012).
- Potentially traumatic, in so far as those directly exposed to them have 'experienced, witnessed, or been confronted with an event or events that involve actual or threatened death or serious injury, or a threat to the physical integrity of oneself or others' (American Psychiatric Association 2000). Heroes may be those who take the 'fight' rather than the 'flight' option in disasters, rushing in to save others at the expense of themselves. In addition to generating physical and psychological reactions during immediate impact, the traumatic nature of such events continues to generate psychosocial effects in the following days and weeks. For those whose natural instinct in disaster was to save themselves rather than others survivor guilt may be compounded by the lavish praise being bestowed on the selflessness of heroes.
- Large-scale community events with likely ripple effects and impacts. The community effects of disaster are described by the sociologist Kai Erikson in the aftermath of the Buffalo Creek flooding disaster, 1973. His classic ethnographic account gives a powerful description of the effects of collective trauma which he describes as a blow to the basic tissues of social life that damages the bonds attaching people together and impairs the prevailing sense of communality.
- Rob Gordon (2009) has analysed further the social processes and dynamics that transpire within a community when a disaster strikes. He describes how emerging distinctions and differences between individuals can cause cleavage planes, severing the fabric of social support systems and causing tension and conflict during recovery stages. Singling out and rewarding some individuals as heroic may create or reinforce unhelpful or unintended hierarchies of worthiness

exacerbating group or community tensions, for example, where some individual acts or actors are formally commended with awards, while others are not.

- Public and political events in which every detail, decision and action by those involved as victims, survivors, witnesses and responders, as well as the reactions of those mourning and bereaved, may be observed, scrutinised and evaluated. Legal accountability for actions in disasters, both individual and corporate, may be examined through lengthy processes and procedures such as inquests, public inquiries, and health and safety investigations. Far from praising the risk-taking behaviour and morality of heroes, legal judgements and disciplinary procedures may take a rather more negative view of such actions.

Disaster Behaviour: Bringing Out the Best in People

Social scientists have spent decades reviewing human reactions and responses to disasters as part of their studies of individual and collective behaviour. Their contribution is a reminder of the importance of ensuring the needs of people are at the heart of emergency planning, response and recovery strategies. Working with emergency managers, they seek to make sure emergency plans and procedures are appropriate and successful by being based on experience and evidence about how people typically behave and respond in the impact and aftermath phases of disaster. Furthermore, their work plays an important role in demystifying and debunking the erroneous myths and beliefs often perpetuated by media and other, often partial, reports of disaster behaviour.

Examples of disaster myths include the notions that disasters produce wide scale, counterproductive and antisocial behaviour such as panic, social disorganisation and looting. This is not to say that such phenomena do not exist, but rather that reports about their prevalence often tend to be exaggerated by the media. In fact, evidence from across different kinds of disaster and societies suggests that on the whole, endangered public and disaster victims respond and adapt well during and after disasters (Tierney et al. 2006:58).

Contrary to the classic notion of the 'disaster syndrome' – a zombie-like condition that renders disaster victims as hapless and helpless (Quarantelli and Dynes 1970) – social scientific research has also highlighted that, at least in the immediate aftermath of disasters, community resilience and unity, strengthening of social ties, self-help, heightened initiative, altruism and prosocial behaviour more often prevail (Auf der Heide 2004).

An example of prosocial, positive responses to disaster was the way in which the people of Oklahoma reacted in the aftermath of the bombing of the Murrah Building on 19 April 1995.

Behaviour later described as 'selfless acts of heroism' (Coats 2011) included local citizens and members of the emergency services running towards the disaster scene to rescue survivors immediately after the bombing rather than away from the building.

This behaviour and other examples led to the term 'The Oklahoma Standard' being coined to define a new level of caring during and after disasters:

> When a need for blood was broadcast, it had to be followed by an advisory to stay home, because more people lined up than were needed. When an announcement was made that work boots were needed at the site, workers pulled up and took off their boots and left them. First responders from out of town found that they could not go to a restaurant and pay for their own meals. Either the restaurant owner would refuse their money or another diner had already covered the ticket. The legend of the "Oklahoma Dollar" is based upon a first responder commenting that he was leaving Oklahoma with the same dollar he had when he arrived because, during his entire stay in Oklahoma, he had been unable to spend that dollar. (The Oklahoma City National Memorial 2013)

The behaviour exhibited during and after this incident was not unusual for large-scale mass fatality incidents. Reinforcing the themes of Erikson and Gordon above, Zunin and Myers (2000) refer to a 'honeymoon' phase reflecting a common aspect of community responses in disaster. They describe this as following on from a rescue or 'heroic' phase where people may risk their own safety to save others, including strangers.

Heroism, Self-Sacrifice and Disasters

The association between life-saving actions and heroism dates back as far as Greek mythology where heroes (and heroines) were depicted as courageous characters displaying the will for self-sacrifice for some greater good of all humanity. They were often venerated as demigods, and although today's heroes may not quite be worshipped in the traditional sense, the cult of the hero personality may seem close to adulation at times. Today, heroism remains associated with moral excellence and positive qualities such as nobility, bravery, and fortitude (Bloomsbury 1993).

Although the popular meaning and application of notions of heroism to disaster-related behaviour has been somewhat stretched in contemporary popular culture,[2] it still tends to be associated with positive moral qualities, meritorious life-saving endeavours and exceptional acts of self-sacrifice. In 2015, seven crews within Staffordshire Fire and Rescue Service received their Chief Officer's certificate of commendation after their work rescuing survivors of a rollercoaster crash at Alton Towers Theme Park. The award is given to people who have placed their lives at reasonable risk while saving others or whose actions have saved lives. Meanwhile, three medics who ignored health and safety considerations at the same incident to rescue trapped and seriously injured individuals were given a Pride of Britain Award (BBC News 2015b). Examples where heroes have been identified by the media and praised for their actions also include the extreme risk-taking as part of initial rescue

---

[2] For example, an online game produced by the US Department of Homeland Security/FEMA claims to equip players with all the information, tips and resources needed to prepare them to be 'a real-life Disaster Hero' in the aftermath of natural disaster or a man-made disaster. (http://www.disasterhero.com/)

efforts in responses to terrorist incidents in Oklahoma City (1995), New York City (2001), London (2005), Glasgow (2007), Boston (2013) and Paris (2015).

The hero label is commonly applied by journalists and members of the public as part of telling the story and a simplistic media discourse about good (heroes) and bad (blameworthy) people in the aftermath of disasters. It is interesting to see how the media return to familiar themes and phrases in telling stories from one disaster to another. The notion of a 'human bridge', for example, used to describe a British man helping fellow passengers to safety during the sinking of the Costa Concordia in 2012 was the same description applied to another British hero during the sinking of a ferry off Zeebrugge in 1987 (United Press International 1987; Fricker 2012; BBC News 2007; Kent Online 2012).

Beyond the media, academic reviews also include references and analyses of the heroic actions of individuals associated with disasters, rescue and response (e.g. Lois 1999). Levinson (2002) raises the question of the appropriateness of this. Analysing Israeli news media coverage of bombing incidents over two consecutive days in Jerusalem and Haifa in 2001, he critiques the accuracy of initial accounts including dramatic reports of heroism which formed a key element of the coverage. Drawing on the work of others, he reflects on how accounts of heroism are part of what makes disaster stories 'newsworthy':

> Levinson (2002) states that the selection of obtrusive incidents for reporting by newspapers depends critically on editorial perceptions of what kinds of event appeal to the public imagination. Stories about disasters have much to offer in this respect, as they can be dramatic, emotive and awe inspiring. Also they furnish numerous opportunities for reporting personal dramas and heroic rescues, for indulging the public's apparent fascination with horrific events, and for satiating the apparent wish of many people to experience vicariously the suffering and tragedy of others.

The Disaster Hero: A Good News Angle on a Bad News Story

In addition to raising the important question of whether accounts of heroism in disasters are accurate such commentary helps explain why references to heroism may be so prolific in disaster reporting. Accounts of heroism are eminently newsworthy, satisfying the thirst for a good news angle on a bad news story. Not only this, disaster heroism is 'newsworthy' in the classic sense because it involves unexpected and dramatic events and includes a human interest perspective with which the audience may be able to personally connect and find meaning (Galtung and Ruge 1965).

The newsworthiness of the disaster hero may even contribute to circumstances where the hero becomes the story in itself, well beyond reports of emergency rescue or response that initially impelled an individual or individuals into the limelight. A cult of personality may arise, established and propagated by the mass media and social media, whereby a hero's identity and actions take on a dynamic life and significance of their own, potentially in place of truth, accuracy or proportionality.

An example of this is John Smeaton, a baggage handler at Glasgow International Airport, who was involved in helping to thwart a terrorist attack there in 2007. When terrorists drove a burning jeep filled with explosives into the airport entrance, Smeaton helped to wrestle one of the attackers to the ground. He was subsequently hailed a hero for having stood up to the terrorists and received a string of awards and positive affirmations. A John Smeaton Appreciation Society was set up on Facebook hailing him a 'hero for our time' and a tribute website received 500,000 hits in its first 48 h. Smeaton gave television interviews which were broadcast worldwide, and over the following months, he was invited to meet a number of senior political figures including the prime minister, and the New York City Mayor Michael R. Bloomberg. His awards included the CNN Everyday Superhero Award, a Daily Mirror Pride of Britain Award and a Queen's Gallantry Medal.

A year later, reports began to circulate in the national press that Smeaton's involvement in the incident had been exaggerated and that others who had done more to restrain the attackers had not been recognised with awards such as the Queen's Gallantry Medal. Smeaton was branded a fake and found himself on the receiving end of negative media attention (BBC 2008). Interviewed 5 years after the incident, he described the impact of being assigned a hero label:

> It was absolutely crazy. I just did what I thought I had to do.... I went to help the police officer. Before I knew it, I am thrust into the limelight. I had everybody chasing after me. To be honest, I didn't know what way to turn, what to do.... It was very difficult. I am a normal guy, and all of a sudden I am on the front page of newspapers, on international news programmes. You don't know which way to turn. It was unbelievable.

Heroism as Resistance to Terrorism

A symbolic aspect of Smeaton's 'heroism' was the sense that his actions not only thwarted a violent act but spoke for the wider public, nationally and internationally, in resisting the fear and threat generated by terrorism. In a television news interview days after the incident, watched by millions around the world, a journalist asked him what message he would give to any future terrorist who tried to launch an attack. Smeaton replied:

> They can try and come to Britain, and they'll try and disrupt us any way they want, but the British people have been under a lot worse things than this and we always stand proud and (if) you come to Glasgow, Glasgow doesn't accept this, do you know what I mean, this is Glasgow, you know, so we'll set about you. (STV 2007)

In this setting, heroism represented of resilience and defiance against the threat and vulnerability caused by international terrorism. Perhaps faith in the power of heroes in the face of violent and traumatic scenes affirms the social belief that goodness and goodwill prevails over threats to safety and social harmony. The need to identify people as heroes may be an unconscious response to the sense of collective threat posed by the terrorists and a need to affirm the belief that most people are good, rather than bad, in a world that really is a safe place most of the time.

While at its roots there have been political connotations attached to legends of heroism and personality cults, equating heroic spontaneous reactions with political resistance to terrorism may be confusing. Similarly, in defining heroism, there is an important distinction to be made between suffering injury during disaster and taking explicit actions taken to save the lives of others as an incident unfolds. It becomes problematic if survival per se becomes a reason to call someone a hero.

In the days after the Boston bombings, 2013, some media reports applied the 'hero' label more generally to people present at the scene as victims, bystanders and responders. The term seemed to be being liberally used to distinguish between non-perpetrators and those who perpetrated the deliberate act of violence. The inference here was that 'heroism' is associated with innocence and with resistance to evil and the terrorists' intention.

One seriously injured survivor, Jeff Bauman, attracted extensive media attention for his 'heroism' which has been associated both with surviving and with trying to help the authorities identify the perpetrators by giving them a description:

> We're just so proud of him', said his boss Kevin Horst. 'We do consider him a hero, both for what he did for law enforcement, whatever role he played in that, but more importantly, he's a hero for how he's handling this time. He's got such a great attitude. (WCVB 2013)

The local news media reported how the 'Boston bombing hero' was receiving dozens of letters each day from people moved by his story. His colleagues created 'Team Bauman' T-shirts, and one news report stated that he had received more than $600,000 in donations for his medical bills over the previous week (Peterson 2013).

Everyone's a Hero, but Some Are More Heroic than Others

In the immediate aftermath of the Boston bombings, much media focus was on identifying and detaining the perpetrators, and so it is understandable that efforts to assist the authorities was greatly appreciated within the wider community. Loosely aligning notions, heroism to crime reporting in these circumstance however is unhelpful because, again, it blurs distinctions, in this case between acts of genuine self-sacrifice and civic duty. Furthermore, it makes the decision to formally recognise truly heroic behaviour more difficult since everyone involved may potentially be identified as a hero.

Alternatively, calling everyone caught up in or responding to disaster a hero may be an attractive prospect for some people since it prevents differentiation and the idea of some heroes being singled out by the media as being more heroic than others. John Smeaton, for example, later acknowledged that others too had acted bravely during the Glasgow attack, not just him, adding: 'They all should be recognised for their efforts and behaviour instead of debating who did the most. It should not be turned into a competition' (Fraser 2012).

Another example of this sentiment was displayed by Thomas Barrett, a patrolman in the Boston Police described by Time Magazine as 'A Hero Among Heroes' for acting on his instinct and training in assisting injured people in the bombings. Barrett's response to the attribution reflected the instinct to label everyone involved as heroes, not just himself, as Time Magazine reported:

> It's a moment of valour he won't soon forget. Barrett borrows a quote about a character from Stephen Ambrose's *Band of Brothers* to describe the experience: "His grandson asked him if he was a hero in the war, and he said, 'No, I wasn't. But I served in the company of heroes.'" Last Monday, Barrett thought similarly. "That day, everybody from my station was a hero. Everybody from the police department was a hero. And at that point, everybody in the city was a hero". (Time Magazine 2013)

The Costs of Heroism: Intrusion and Survivor Guilt

Today, disaster scenes are beamed into our living rooms including breaking news stories covering every aspect of the unfolding drama. More than ever before, disasters have become public events in the sense of actions, reactions and behavioural responses being captured, recorded, reviewed and replayed through social and other media. The cost of this may be uninvited intrusions into privacy. For some people caught up in this media analysis, enduring coverage renders them unable to escape public attention, exposure and scrutiny. This may be all the more unwelcome during at particularly sensitive times such as the fraught emotional aftermath of a traumatic experience.

It is not unusual for those to whom the hero label is attributed to express reluctance and to resist or deflect media attention. Associating their actions with implications of extraordinary qualities and goodness may feel inappropriate or unfair. Examples of this following the Boston bombing include:

- A man photographed carrying a woman to safety after the explosions who, when interviewed, said: 'While I appreciate the interest in hearing our perspective on today's horrific events, the spotlight should remain firmly on the countless individuals – first responders, medics, EMTs, runners who crossed the finish line and kept on running straight to give blood, and the countless civilians – who did whatever they could to save lives. They were the true heroes'.
- An active-duty service member photographed wrapping the red shirt he wore during the Marathon around the bloody leg of a man at the blast site. His reluctance to be identified led to his being referred to as 'the man who gave the shirt off his back' (NBC News 2013).

Focussing on heroism can distract from the true horrors of confronting mass death and injury. Meanwhile, for those whose natural instinct and reaction during disaster was to save themselves and flee from danger, notions of heroism may later feed powerful reactions of survivor guilt. Writing a few weeks after the Boston bombing, journalist Beth Teitell (2013) recorded how, since the attack, many of the wounded have shared their stories with the public. But, she adds, 'in private, some uncounted number of runners and spectators are suffering from feelings of intense guilt because when violence struck, they didn't dash in to help. Instead, they made sure their own loved ones were safe amid the harrowing chaos – or fled the danger to make sure they would survive to care for their families'.

Teitell interviewed Jane Blansfield Finch, a clinical social worker and Red Cross volunteer about their reactions. Finch suggested that even though many anointed as heroes said they did not deserve the honour, the public veneration of those who jump to help in a disaster serves a greater purpose because it encourages altruism. At the same time, she acknowledged that there is a downside: 'It puts pressure on people to think, "If I'm not out there helping strangers, am I worthwhile?"' (Teitell 2013).

Emergency Service Responders as Heroes

For members of the emergency services, there can be a strong sense that risk-taking comes with the job, but the exceptional conditions associated with disaster response and recovery has particular implications for both their role and subsequent recognition of their actions in relation to heroism. When emergency responders become identified as disaster heroes, stories highlighting their personal circumstances and subsequent lives are invariably newsworthy, especially if they can be linked to a salacious or sensationalist storyline (e.g. Camber 2011; Stritof 2013). Unsurprisingly, for example, much media coverage was given internationally to Bryce Reed, the paramedic first hailed a hero for helping save victims of the fertiliser plant explosion in West, Texas, and later charged with the federal charge of possessing an explosive device.

After the London Bombings on 7 July 2005, 23 members of emergency teams and transport workers who helped victims of the attacks were formally recognised in the Queen's New Year Honours list in 2006 (BBC News 2005). Many others who behaved heroically on that day were not so recognised (Addley 2011). And in contrast to this period, where certain heroic acts were formally recognised and publicly praised, aspects of the emergency response as a whole were later criticised, both in the report of the London Assembly in 2006 and in the inquests conducted during 2011 into why 52 innocent people died.

Although the emergency response on 7 July was commended on the whole, such intense public scrutiny and elements of criticism during the lengthy subsequent legal procedures must have had an impact on all involved in the emergency response, including those who may have felt a sense of falling 'from hero to zero'. It is important that psychological, social and organisational support is made available for responders during these later, longer-term phases following disaster as inevitable legal procedures take their course. The impact of events and their appraisal may be no less significant at these points.

Tributes to Fallen Heroes

When first responders lose their lives during disaster response, the impact on families, public service organisations and the wider community is painfully felt and especially poignant, even more so when there is multiple loss. Tributes by key political and national figures in the aftermath of such events often make specific reference to their bravery and heroism.

An example of this is the following comment made by Sanford Coats, the US Attorney for the Western District of Oklahoma, in remembering the tenth anniversary of the tragic events on 11 September 2001 and 19 April 1995:

> Just like the morning of September 11, brave Oklahoma fire fighters, medical personnel, and peace officers risked their lives by going into a burning, unstable building in *selfless acts of heroism* to rescue survivors. Indeed, one first responder gave the ultimate sacrifice in an effort to rescue survivors, becoming one of the 168 casualties of the bomb. (Sanford Coates; parentheses added)

After the explosion at the fertiliser plant in West, Texas (April 2013), where 11 of the 144 fatalities were firefighters, the news media made specific reference to the fact that most of the deaths were first responders and, as with other disasters where multiple members of the emergency services are killed, the mourning rituals and memorials received special media coverage (Fernandez 2013)). In an article entitled 'Heroes in West, Texas explosion honoured', *USA Today* reported on President Obama travelling to the town to speak at the memorial service for those killed in the explosion and ordering flags at government building to be lowered to half-mast in honour of the victims (USA Today 2013).

Heroism, Common Sense and Common Safety

If heroism is about exceptional or extraordinary behaviour, should it be applied to the ordinary work of members of the emergency services? Clearly, distinctions are made between the usual and exceptional work of emergency responders when bravery awards are given to recognise particular acts of merit as opposed to actions that are more run of the mill. Notions of heroism as reflecting moral virtue also raise important questions about what kinds of attitudes and behaviours are right, appropriate and desirable in those exceptional environments, where many lives are at risk or in situations where the lives of some may be put at greater risk through potential life-saving actions for others. Such questions fall within the remit of health and safety law and practice, but there are broader philosophical and practical issues to consider:

> There is (also) a need to stimulate a debate about risk in society to ensure that everyone has a much better understanding of risk and its management. (Loftstedt 2011:6)

In the UK, discussions about heroism in the emergency services have been prompted by just such a debate and developments in health and safety. In 2010, the UK

Government commissioned a review by Lord Young of the Operation of Health and Safety Laws (HM Government 2010). While the driver was to reduce bureaucracy, confusion and fears of an increasingly litigious 'compensation culture', the review also focussed on activities of members of the emergency services and the implications for acts of heroism. It outlined the responsibility of employees under health and safety legislation to take reasonable care of themselves and others, but it added that the nature of jobs within the emergency services means individuals may occasionally put themselves at risk to save the life of someone else. Where this happens, stated the report, the last thing that should be contemplated is a prosecution for non-compliance with health and safety legislation. Lord Young stated:

> Where an unfortunate incident occurs and an officer puts him or herself at risk in the line of their duty to protect the public, I take the view that it would not be in the public interest to take action and investigate under health and safety laws.

However, Lord Young also recognised that there was some ambiguity in such cases and a need for greater certainty in this important area (2010:35). Indeed, this is illustrated in his comments further on in the report:

> It is important to recognise that individuals have personal choices to make and they may choose not to put themselves at unreasonable risk. However, those officers who go the extra mile and put themselves in harm's way to protect the public should continue to be recognised and rewarded for their bravery. (2010:36)

The report thus recommended that 'police officers and fire-fighters should not be at risk of investigation or prosecution under health and safety legislation when engaged in the course of their duties if they have put themselves at risk as a result of committing a heroic act' and invited the Health and Safety Executive (HSE), the Association of Chief Police Officers and Crown Prosecution Service to consider further guidance to put this into effect (2010:36).

Balancing Operational and Health and Safety Duties

This focus on risk, health and safety within emergency response came at a significant moment in the UK. In the preceding years, the challenging nature and extremely dangerous environments in which firefighters and other emergency responders have to work had been highlighted by a series of serious and fatal incidents which had exposed emergency responders to personal risk in the course of their attempts to rescue victims. At the same time, the actions and risk assessments of responders were coming under some criticism by investigators, the media and the public, including bereaved families. The incidents and investigations included:

- The London Bombings, 2005, which killed 52 people and four terrorists, and where the response of the emergency services was reviewed and critiqued both through the inquest and a review by the London Assembly (Greater London Authority 2006).

- The death of a woman trapped in a mine shaft in 2008 whose rescue was inhibited for over 6 h. The fatal accident inquiry concluded Mrs Hume may have lived if emergency services – and the fire service in particular – had removed her sooner. The sheriff's ruling criticised procedural failings which led to the delay, and said senior officers on the scene 'rigidly stood by their operational guidelines' (Carrell 2011; BBC News March 2012).
- The Cumbria shootings, 2010, in which 12 members of the public lost their lives and a further 11 people were seriously injured. A peer review of the emergency response by the Assistant Chief Constable of West Mercia Police concluded that there were differing 'risk thresholds' between the services and that the interoperability between the police and ambulance service needed to be improved (Chesterman 2011).
- A fatal fire at a warehouse in Warwickshire, 2007, where four firefighters lost their lives (BBC 2010). Warwickshire County Council was fined £30,000 after pleading guilty to a health and safety charge. Three fire service managers were prosecuted for manslaughter by gross negligence. After all were found not guilty, the Chief Fire Officer condemned the decision to press criminal charges against them (BBC News 7 December 2012).

As a result of these and other incidents, the Health and Safety Executive (HSE) began working with senior leaders of the police and fire services to clarify a number of complex and interrelated issues. Their aim was to avoid a risk-averse culture, provide mechanisms for ensuring early and wide learning from incidents and set out the expectations on the services in relation to the management of dynamic and often dangerous situations.

Redefining 'Heroic Acts' of Emergency Responders

Endorsing the recommendations of the Young report, the Health and Safety Executive, Association of Chief Police Officers, Police Authorities and Fire and Rescue Authorities worked together to identify how a balance could be struck between high-risk operational duties and the health and safety of themselves and others. The result has been the issuing of statements and further guidance for both the Police Service and the Fire and Rescue Authorities clarifying the balance between operational and health and safety duties in the emergency services and clarifying the meaning and consequences of acts deemed heroic (HSE 2009; HSE 2010).

In relation to the fire service, for example, the HSE has clarified its interpretation and actions relating to 'heroism' as follows:

'HSE will view the actions of individual fire-fighters as heroic when:

- it is clear that they have decided to act entirely of their own volition;
- they have put themselves at risk to protect the public or colleagues; and
- the individuals' actions were not likely to have put other officers or members of the public at serious risk.

In the event of HSE being notified of a serious incident, inspectors may need to make initial enquiries about the nature of the incident and may need to conduct an investigation of the Service's operational arrangements and management of health and safety. If, during this investigation, it becomes clear, however, that the incident involved an act of heroism by individual fire-fighters, then the HSE will not investigate the actions of the individuals in order to take any action against them'. (HSE 2010)

Concluding Comments

There is likely to be much interest in the UK in the application of this guidance in the event of it having to be applied following future emergencies and disasters. More broadly, and with reference to the themes explored in this chapter, members of the UK Emergency Services and the wider public might benefit from a more informed understanding and debate about the meaning and implications of notions of 'heroism', particularly in the context of extreme events.

In the USA too, where a different cultural and legal environment exists for considering issues around notions of heroism, litigation, and health and safety guidance exists (IAFF/NIOSH 2013), and further debate has begun about the context and consequences of 'heroism', the actions of emergency responders and the implications of their actions on both families and responders themselves (Nicol 2013). Ultimately, such reflections may also contribute to our thinking and expectations around good, worthy and commendable behaviour in more ordinary circumstances.

The characteristic of genuine heroism is its persistency. All men have wandering impulses, fits and starts of generosity. But when you have resolved to be great, abide by yourself, and do not weakly try to reconcile yourself with the world. The heroic cannot be the common, nor the common the heroic. (Ralph Waldo Emerson 1841)

References

Addley, E. (2011). 7/7: How victims and heroes were made with a terrible randomness. *The Guardian*. http://www.guardian.co.uk/uk/2011/jan/27/7-7-bombings-victims.

American Psychiatric Association. (2000). *Diagnostic and statistical manual of mental disorders* (Revised 4th ed.). Washington, DC: Author.

Auf der Heide, E. (2004). Common misconceptions about disasters: Panic, the "disaster syndrome," and looting, O'Leary, M. (Ed.), (2004). *The first 72 hours: A community approach to disaster preparedness*. Lincoln (Nebraska): iUniverse Publishing.

BBC News. (2015a, August). Paris train attack heroes awarded with France's top honour, August 24, 2015. http://www.bbc.co.uk/news/world-europe-34038055.

BBC News. (2015b, September). Alton Towers Smiler crash bravery award for 'rule-breakers', September 24, 2015. http://www.bbc.co.uk/news/uk-england-34350586.

BBC News. (2010, December). Timeline: Warwickshire fire-fighter deaths. *BBC News*, December 7, 2012. http://www.bbc.co.uk/news/uk-england-coventry-warwickshire-16651345.

BBC News. (2012, March). Alison Hume inquiry: Mineshaft rescue 'lacked focus', March 29, 2012. http://www.bbc.co.uk/news/uk-scotland-glasgow-west-17552330.

BBC News. (2008). Airport hero rejects 'fake' claim, Sunday, 16 March 2008, 13:49 GMT. http://news.bbc.co.uk/1/hi/scotland/glasgow_and_west/7299436.stm

BBC News. (2007). 1987: Zeebrugge heroes honoured, On this Day, December 31, 1997. http://news.bbc.co.uk/onthisday/hi/dates/stories/december/31/newsid_2560000/2560075.stm.

BBC News. (2005). Honours tribute to 7 July workers. *BBC News,* December 31, 2005. http://news.bbc.co.uk/2/hi/uk_news/4569560.stm.

BBC News. (1999). Nothing prepared me for the horror. *BBC News*, October 11, 1999. http://news.bbc.co.uk/1/hi/uk/468271.stm.

Bloomsbury. (1993). *'Hero' – Bloomsbury guide to human thought*. London: Bloomsbury Publishing Ltd. Credo Reference. Web. May 15, 2013; prod.credoreference.com/topic/heroes/pdf.

Camber, R. (2011). 7/7 hero is £100m cocaine kingpin: Fireman among 33 sent to jail as Britain's biggest drugs gang is smashed. http://www.dailymail.co.uk/news/article-1344289/7-7-hero-Simon-Ford--100m-cocaine-kingpin-jailed-police-smash-drug-gang.html#ixzz2Pt73XpMo.

Carrell, S. (2011). Rescue services criticised over death of woman left in mine shaft for six hours. *The Guardian*, November 16, 2011. http://www.guardian.co.uk/uk/2011/nov/16/woman-left-in-mine-shaft.

Chesterman, S. (2011). *Operation Bridge: Peer review into the response of Cumbria Constabulary following the actions of Derrick Bird on 2 June 2010*, Independent Peer Review – Final Report, March 28, 2011. www.cumbria.police.uk/Admin/.../ACC_Chestermans_report.pdf.

Coats, S. (2011). The Oklahoma City Bombing: From national tragedy, we continue through our resilience to work for comfort, strength, peace, hope and serenity', U.S. Attorney for the Western District of Oklahoma. (http://www.justice.gov/usao/briefing_room/ns/oklahoma_city.html).

Emerson, R. W. (1841). *Essays and english traits*. Vol. V. The harvard classics. New York: P.F. Collier & Son, 1909–14; Bartleby.com, 2001. http://www.bartleby.com/5/107.html. (May 17, 2013).

Fernandez, M. (2013). A Texas town mourns the first responders who paid with their lives. *The New York Times*, April 20, 2013. http://www.nytimes.com/2013/04/21/us/in-texas-mourning-first-responders-who-paid-with-their-lives.html?pagewanted=all&_r=0.

Fraser, G. (2012). John Smeaton: From Glasgow Airport terror attack hero to fish farmer, June 30, 2012. http://local.stv.tv/glasgow/magazine/108635-john-smeaton-from-glasgow-airport-terror-attack-hero-to-fish-farmer/.

Fricker, M. (2012). Costa Concordia: Hero British teenager made himself into human ladder to save passengers. *Daily Mirror*, Januray 17, 2012. http://www.mirror.co.uk/news/uk-news/costa-concordia-hero-british-teenager-158783.

Galtung, J., & Ruge, M. (1965). The structure of foreign news: The presentation of the Congo, Cuba and Cyprus crises in four Norwegian newspapers. *Journal of Peace Research, 2*(1), 64–90.

Gordon, R. (2009). Community impact of disaster and community recovery. InPsych, Australian Psychological Society, April 2009. http://www.psychology.org.au/inpsych/community_impact/#s3.

Greater London Authority. (2006). Report of the 7 July review committee, London, June 2006. http://www.london.gov.uk/mayor-assembly/london-assembly/publications/report-7-july-review-committee.

H M Coroner. (2012). Coroner's inquest into the London Bombings of 7 July 2005, Judicial Communications Office. http://webarchive.nationalarchives.gov.uk/20120216072438/http://7julyinquests.independent.gov.uk/.

H M Government. (2010). *Common sense, common safety*. London: Cabinet Office.

HSE. (2010). Striking the balance between operational and health and safety duties in the fire and rescue service. *Crown Copyright*. http://www.hse.gov.uk/services/fire/heroism.htm.

HSE. (2009). Striking the balance between operational and health and safety duties in the police service. *Crown Copyright*. http://www.hse.gov.uk/services/police/duties.pdf.

International Association of Fire Fighters/National Institute of Occupational Safety and Health (IAFF/NIOSH). (2013). Suggested Guidance for Supervisors at Disaster Rescue Sites. Washington DC: IAFF/NIOSH. Retrieved from http://www.iaff.org/hs/Alerts/NIOSHdisaster.asp.

Kent Online. (2012). Andrew Parker – The human stepping stone, The HFE Tragedy 25 Years on, Accessed 8 Apr 2013. http://www.kentonline.co.uk/kentonline/home/special_reports/ herald_of_free_enterprise/andrew_parker_-_the_human_step.aspx.

Levinson, J. (2002). Israeli news media coverage: Bombing near Zion Square, Jerusalem. *Disaster Prevention and Management, online, 11*(1). Accessed April 20, 2013.

Loftstedt, R. (2011). Reclaiming health and safety for all: An independent review of health and safety legislation, Presented to Parliament by the Secretary of State for Work and Pensions by Command of Her Majesty, November 2011, CM 8219, Crown Copyright.

Lois, J. (1999). Socialization to heroism: Individualism and collectivism in a voluntary search and rescue group. *Social Psychology Quarterly, 62*(2), 17–135.

NBC News. (2013). Amid the chaos and carnage in Boston, heroes emerge. http://usnews.nbcnews. com/_news/2013/04/16/17780108-amid-the-chaos-and-carnage-in-boston-heroes-emerge?lite.

Nicol, S. (2013, August 2). Pa. Firefghters Hear Tearful Message AboutVictim. Firehouse.com News. Retrieved from http://www.firehouse.com/news/11077235/ woman-whose-husband-seriously-hurt-byresponder-asks-dept-not-give-him-heros-funeral.

Peterson, H. (2013). Heartwarming moment bomb hero who lost both his legs gave an 18th birth-day gift to teen who was wounded alongside him. *Mail Online*, 25 April 2013. http://www. dailymail.co.uk/news/article-2314195/Jeff-Bauman-Boston-bombings-hero-lost-son-Iraq-describes-emotional-hospital-visit-man-life-famously-saved.html#ixzz2SuGRQjdJ.

Quarantelli, E. L., & Dynes, R. R. (1970). Introduction special issue on organizational and group behaviour in disaster. *The American Behavioral Scientist, 13*(3), 325–330.

Smith, J. (2011). Out of the gloom of disasters shine the heroes who give us all hope. *The Independent*, March 20, 2011. http://www.independent.co.uk/voices/commentators/joan-smith/joan-smith-out-of-the-gloom-of-disasters-shine-the-heroes-who-give-us-all-hope-2246975.html.

Stritof, S. (2013). Cheating heroes: More victims of September 11th. http://marriage.about.com/ cs/infidelity/a/cheatingheroes.htm. Accessed 8 Apr 2013.

STV. (2007). Glasgow airport attack: John Smeaton becomes a worldwide celebrity. *STV Glasgow*. http://local.stv.tv/glasgow/magazine/108635-john-smeaton-from-glasgow-airport-terror-attack-hero-to-fish-farmer/. Accessed 17 May 2013.

Teitell, B. (2013). Some agonize over fleeing Marathon bombing scene. *The Boston Globe*, May 09, 2013. http://www.bostonglobe.com/lifestyle/style/2013/05/08/boston-marathon-heroes-are-lauded-some-who-didn-rush-help-grapple-with-guilt/SNUKlSFLDMKTmz3Sen69dP/ story.html.

The Oklahoma City National Memorial Foundation. (2013). The Oklahoma Standard, Oklahoma City National Memorial and Museum. http://www.oklahomacitynationalmemorial.org/second-ary.php?section=6&catid=165. Accessed 2013.

Tierney, K., Bevc, C., & Kuligowski, E. (2006). Metaphors matter: Disaster myths, media frames, and their consequences in hurricane Katrina. *The Annals of the American Academy of Political and Social Science, 604*, 57–81.

Time Magazine. (2013). A hero among heroes: A Boston Cop's story at the marathon. http://nation.time.com/2013/04/22/a-hero-among-heroes-a-boston-cops-story-at-the-marathon/#ixzz2StoEUom9.

TNT Magazine. (2012, January 17). British cruise ship hero survivor acted as 'human bridge'. http://www. tntmagazine.com/travel/news/british-cruise-ship-hero-survivor-acted-as-uhuman-bridgeu.

United Press International. (1987). Lanky Banker's human bridge saved 20 on Ferry, March 10, 1987.

USA Today. (2013). Heroes in West, Texas explosion honoured. *USA Now video, USA Today*. http://www.usatoday.com/videos/news/usanow/2013/04/25/2112287/.

WCVB. (2013). Communities rally support for Boston bombing hero, April 27, 2013. http:// www.wcvb.com/news/local/metro/communities-rally-support-for-boston-bombing-hero/-/11971628/19923962/-/jqqoolz/-/index.html.

Yokota, T., & Yamada, T. (2012). Heroes of Japan's nuclear disaster all but forgotten, The Daily Beast, *Newsweek*, March 4, 2012 http://www.thedailybeast.com/newsweek/2012/03/04/ heroes-of-japan-s-nuclear-disaster-all-but-forgotten.html.

Zunin, L. M. & Myers, D. (2000). *Training manual for human service workers in major disasters* (2nd ed.) Washington, DC: Department of Health and Human Services, Substance Abuse and Mental Health Services Administration, Centre for Mental Health Services; DHHS Publication No. ADM 90–538.

Dr. Anne Eyre (BA Hons, PhD) is a sociologist and independent consultant specialising in psychosocial aspects of major incidents, emergency planning and disaster management. Her work focusses on the ensuring that the needs of people are at the heart of contingency planning, emergency response and recovery. Anne is a Fellow of the Winston Churchill Memorial Trust, and in 2006, she spent time in New York and New Jersey examining community support strategies after the terrorist attacks in September 2001, including the support by and for New York's emergency responder communities after 9/11. She is on several editorial boards including the International Fire Service Journal of Leadership and Management, and in 2013, she was awarded the Granito Award for Excellence in Fire Leadership and Management Research. Her latest book is Collective Conviction: The Story of Disaster Action, with Pamela Dix, Liverpool University Press, Liverpool (2014) https://www.amazon.co.uk/Collective-Conviction-Disaster-Action/dp/1781381232. Contact: anne.eyre@traumatraining.com.

Chapter 9
Older Firefighters: A Problem to Be Managed or a Resource to Be Valued?

Anita Pickerden

Introduction

The UK Fire and Rescue Service (FRS) (along with all other parts of the public sector) has experienced profound changes, many of which have had a direct effect upon the working lives of its workforce.

To take account of the ageing population and the pressure upon pensions, additional legislation has extended the State Pension Age and also removed the Default Retirement Age so that older workers are not obliged to finish work at 60–65, and eventually both male and female retirees will receive their state pension at 67, 68 or even older. While some FRS employers are becoming more aware of their general obligations towards older workers, their willingness to provide policies to address the specific needs of older firefighters is not yet universal.

In the past, the firefighters' pension arrangements made it uneconomical for any firefighter to continue working for more than 30 years, but this no longer applies. The abolition of the Default Retirement Age and the gender equalisation rules have paved the way for the proposed pension changes for firefighters which were laid before parliament at the end of October 2014, despite considerable resistance from the Fire Brigades Union. Politics aside, it is clear that the Fire and Rescue Service employers will be faced with an ageing workforce over the next few years, and many of those employees will be operational firefighters. On a national basis, changes to the revised pension schemes will see many more people having to work for more years before they receive their occupational and state pensions. The Public Service Pensions Act 2013 set the 'Normal Pension Age' for the 2015 Firefighters' Pension Scheme at age 60. While these changes have impacted the working lives of older firefighters and their supervisors and managers, other political changes have also had an impact and created greater uncertainty for older firefighters.

A. Pickerden (✉)
Worcester Business School, University of Worcester, Worcester, UK
e-mail: anita@pickerden.co.uk

© Springer International Publishing AG 2018
P. Murphy, K. Greenhalgh (eds.), *Fire and Rescue Services*,
DOI 10.1007/978-3-319-62155-5_9

In January 2016, the Government announced that responsibility for the UK FRS would move from the Department of Communities and Local Government (DCLG) to the Home Office, in order to deliver the government's manifesto commitment to deliver greater joint working between the police and fire service. There were already many examples of collaboration between police forces and fire services across the country, including Northamptonshire, where a programme had been sharing training, premises and operations teams across all three emergency services. In Durham, Tri-service Community Safety Responders were trained to act as PCSOs, retained firefighters and community first responders (i.e. volunteer, on-call NHS ambulance personnel). Many of the existing collaborations were an attempt to save money in the light of continuing public sector cuts. This was by no means the first change in governance; originally, the FRS had been regulated and inspected by the Home Office from 1947 until 2001 when it was transferred to the Department for Transport, Local Government and the Regions (now disbanded). Then, in May 2002, it was transferred to the Office of the Deputy Prime Minister (ODPM) which was changed in July 2006 to the Department of Communities and Local Government and now back to the Home Office.

Another change announced by the government in January 2016 was that police and crime commissioners (PCCs), and in some cases, the new regional combined authority mayors would be able to bid to take over employment responsibilities for Fire and Rescue services. The minister for policing, fire, criminal justice and victims, Mike Penning, made the case for realignment, joint working and shared premises as being cost effective and beneficial to the public. Many in the FRS were concerned at the time that the good will and trust enjoyed by firefighters might be diminished by closer connection with the Police. This concern would appear to have been allayed with promises that reorganisation at the top of the organisations would not mean that the two organisations were to be merged. The Policing and Crime Bill 2016 was passed in the Commons and is due for scrutiny in the House of Lords from 14 September 2016. The very different approaches by the Police and Fire Services regarding retirement age has caused concern to firefighters. While the FRS expects firefighters to work until 60, Police have employment contracts that enable them to 'retire' police officers at 50 for economic reasons. This confusion has to be addressed by the PCC and/or Combined Authority Mayors in due course.

Theoretical Background (Life Course Analysis)

Using the theoretical framework of life-course analysis as a starting point, the traditional career story of a firefighter in the English FRS was to join the service in their late teens or early twenties, spend a considerable number of years attached to a crew, possibly gain promotion and retire after 30 years' employment, usually in their early 50s. Many firefighters joined because they already had relatives in the fire service and so were aware of the shift and watch systems. Fire Service Pensions, which are governed by statute, provided a generous lump sum and monthly pension, although many retired firefighters went on to work in new careers, or set up their own business. Some even returned to their original FRS as a non-uniformed employee.

For this research, there were some challenges encountered by using life-course analysis, the five main elements of which are that (a) there is continuity as well as change; (b) the age of a person may be measured as a biological, psychological, social or spiritual age; (c) people interpret the wider world through the lens of their family life; (d) there is often a link between experiences as a child and those in later life; and (e) people can make choices and construct their own life journey by reacting to the opportunities and constraints that face them (Hutchison 2010). In some areas of the research, the life-course perspective was most useful, for example, in contextualising the experience of older firefighters at the hands of their younger colleagues and managers, and in understanding the elements of continuity and change for individuals in a 30-year career pattern. However, other elements were not so helpful, such as whether the decisions made as young people had impacted upon the career choice of firefighters. And the final key element that of making choices according to the circumstances facing the individual at a specific time seemed to be simply stating the obvious. However, it was, on the whole, a useful way of interpreting the individual perceptions and experiences of work of this cohort of older firefighters.

Methods and Data

In the first study, older workers employed by a Metropolitan Fire and Rescue Service were questioned about their attitudes to work as they approached retirement. Although most government literature refers to older workers as being aged over 50, the participants in this study were aged 45 and over, in order to capture the opinions of those firefighters who would have traditionally retired after 30 years' service, that is, in their early 50s. Four hundred questionnaires were sent to all employees aged 45 and over. One hundred and thirteen responses (26%) were received, covering the majority of roles within the FRS, male and female, and spread across the ages of 45–65. Gender and ethnicity followed the national average as indicated by CLG figures (DCLG 2012).

Twenty-five respondents also agreed to answer a series of monthly email questions designed to assess whether their perceptions of the quality of work changed over time. A number of recently retired firefighters also agreed to be interviewed to discuss their careers. The results were then compared with national information gained from a 2008 DCLG survey, and with the results from 25-targeted questionnaires sent to members of what was then known as Networking Women in the Fire Service.

In the second study, a brief questionnaire was sent out to 25 HR directors and managers of the larger English FRS, asking whether they had introduced or planned to introduce policies specifically aimed at their older firefighters. Fourteen FRS responded, most of which had no specific policies in place nor plans to do so.

Challenges Specific to the Fire and Rescue Service

There are a number of perceptions of older firefighters which are influencing the current debate, for example that, as soon as they reach the age of 50, they are no longer mentally or physically fit enough to fight fires and/or rescue people. Many younger workers, when asked their opinion of their older colleagues, suggest that they are too old to learn new skills (particularly using new equipment and technology), very resistant to change and less committed than younger firefighters. Some managers believe that their older firefighters are likely to take more time off sick, take longer to make decisions and are inefficient and less effective. Older workers are seen as blocking the promotion prospects of their younger colleagues and so should be forced to retire, sometimes even earlier than their anticipated pension age (Pritchard and Whiting 2014).

Some of these perceptions are true. It is unlikely that an older firefighter would be able to meet the proposed fitness standards for entry into the fire service, and there is also evidence that ageing tends to affect the speed of decision-making (Beers and Butler 2012), although much of the research involved people aged 60 and over, and the rate of decline was slow.

However, older firefighters are much less likely to take time off due to either injury or sickness, although they do tend to take longer to recover if an accident does occur (Farrow and Reynolds 2012). With regard to issues of loyalty and commitment, this research suggested that firefighters of any age are committed to providing public service, and most older firefighters are more than willing to share their expertise with their younger colleagues, particularly as they are likely to possess much greater operational experience.

But looking at the cultural and commercial value of older firefighters to the FRS, Joe et al. (2013) described them also as 'knowledge workers', possessing subject matter expertise; knowledge about work relationships and social networks; organisational knowledge; institutional memory; knowledge of systems and processes; knowledge of governance; and embedded community awareness. The use of this knowledge would not necessarily have to involve active operational duty in all cases.

Having looked at the perceptions of older firefighters by their younger colleagues, it is only fair to consider the issues that older firefighters themselves reported:

(a) Older firefighters feel they are in the 'sandwich generation' as they may have elderly relatives as well as children to care for (or finance through university). Several reported additional responsibilities looking after grandchildren, and others were looking after sick or disabled partners. Those older workers in second families with young children also found that colleagues did not expect them to need to leave work on time for the school run.

(b) Poor management reduces motivation. It is now very well researched (Kelloway and Barling 2010) that the management abilities of a manager or supervisor will directly affect the wellbeing, motivation and productivity of their staff.

Therefore, those older firefighters who are badly managed will inevitably cause long-term problems for their FRS. Sadly, there is still a bullying culture in a small number of FRSs which will tend to lower motivation and the overall effectiveness of staff.

(c) Older firefighters realised too late that they had made inadequate preparation for their retirement. Many FRSs have reduced the amount of support they provide for planning what to do after retirement from the service and that includes where people might want to be and with whom. Many older firefighters have unrealistic expectations of what they can afford to do when they retire (Moen 2000; Goodwin & O'Connor 2014). For older firefighters, approaching retirement there seems still to be a reluctance to start planning in a timely fashion, even when respondents know that they should have started their planning earlier. Given the general reluctance to carry out forward planning, this could be an area of work for HR personnel who are tasked with employee wellbeing, and this could create longer-term benefits for this target group. US research by Moen (2000) suggests that most retirees regret not saving more/paying off mortgage/not planning and preparing for life after retirement, and this was born out in this study with recent retirees from the Metropolitan FRS. Several found that they were not able to pay off their mortgage and still needed to find employment.

(d) There is a fine balance to be struck between job demands versus job resources, which can impact the performance of older firefighters. There is a well-researched link between (a) job demands and job resources, (b) negative work-home interference and (c) burnout, which includes exhaustion, cynicism and cognitive weariness (Mostert 2011). The job demands include the complexity of the work, additional hazards and physical demands. Resources available to enable a firefighter to carry out the role would include manager and peer support, as well as appropriate training and equipment. Meeting all aspects of the role map as people get older becomes more difficult, especially when Brigade Managers are reluctant to consider minor amendments of the role map for individuals. Recovery time after night shifts increases for older workers, particularly in those FRSs where beds have been removed from stations.

(e) Failure by FRS to fully utilise their skills and knowledge, many older firefighters have undertaken considerable amounts of training and professional development during their careers, yet managers seem to forget this, and much of that valuable knowledge and skill is simply wasted. This is particularly important as the number of incidents and fires has decreased, which reduces the learning opportunities for younger firefighters.

(f) The somewhat dismissive attitude of younger colleagues over an extended period of time can be demotivating or create additional pressure on older firefighters to 'prove' themselves as fit as their colleagues. This can damage morale within a watch or station, which can lower the effectiveness of the older firefighter and could, in extreme, lead to performance management discussions. Rego et al. (2016) note that *Evidence suggests that 'mistaken and irrational' ageism toward older workers prevails in many organizations,* and that these negative beliefs are particularly damaging to both the older workers and to their organisations.

(g) Older firefighters reported feeling trapped by the pension and unable to leave or retire early. This has been a recurring theme, for example, many of the responses in the Department of Communities and Local Government report on Working in the Fire Service (2008) showed that individual firefighters felt that they were no longer happy with their employer, but they did not wish to jeopardise their pension arrangements or felt that they could 'last out' until their retirement date (DCLG 2008).

With regard to concerns about the adequacy of the pension, recent studies by the DWP suggest that 71% of UK workers would be willing to work beyond State Pension Age in order to increase their income. Many others intend to continue working out of interest, either in the same type of work for another employer or in self-employment.

Conclusion and Discussion

The role of the organisation and its managers is crucial in the individual's level of performance; a lack of understanding or empathy for the needs of the individuals in a team can destroy the working relationships within the team as well as damaging the remaining career of an older firefighter. This research suggests that negative beliefs of the abilities of older firefights have increased during the past two decades, compared with the more positive view taken by Hassell and Perrewe (Hassell and Perrewe 1995).

There is an assumption in some organisations that older workers are blocking the progress of younger staff and that they spend the last few years of work just cruising to retirement (Frankel and Picascia 2008). This assumption needs to be challenged, not least because the abolition of the Default Retirement Age means that workers will be able to continue working well beyond their expected retirement date and so their skills and experience have the potential to be a valuable resource for the organisation.

Several older firefighters commented on the lack of empathy and understanding shown to them by their managers and supervisors: although part of this could be due to a general reluctance to interfere in the private lives of team members, not wishing to intrude or to appear nosey. This could easily be dealt with by including issues of planning for retirement in the annual staff appraisal interview; for example, if the person is considering a new training course or promotion, the manager should be able to ask how that would impact on their plans for the next few years. Any squeamishness by the manager would be reduced if a mandatory question was routinely included in the process. Given the changes required by the abolition of the Default Retirement Age, this would be a good time to revisit the annual appraisal questions.

The skills, knowledge and experience of older firefighters are often overlooked or forgotten by their younger managers and supervisors, and the older firefighters reported feeling sidelined as a result. This is partly attributable to reluctance by some older workers to push themselves forward but also to lack of easily accessible personnel records that could give the manager the information they need to know what project to give to which person. A poor system of recording training, qualifications and competences that relies upon the individual employee identifying their own training needs and then recording when they think they have evidenced competence is unlikely to contribute to good management and motivation of older staff.

Many respondents referred to their managers and supervisors showing a complete lack of interest in their abilities despite the fact that the organisation had paid for all of their training and qualifications, and this is demotivating and also a waste of resources, particularly at a time of austerity. A follow-up training workshop for older workers was piloted with the organisation and demonstrated that 1 day's input could help to reverse the feelings of disempowerment and reinvigorate the career plans of older workers in the FRS. This has been successfully duplicated in a number of other organisations and complemented by a shorter session for younger managers to gain more understanding of intergenerational management issues such as motivation and performance management.

The fact that some older workers become disillusioned by their lack of promotion to the higher levels of the organisation, while others are driven by ambition to reach the top at all costs, highlights the need for high levels of management ability. Both groups require careful management to avoid disruption, but it seemed from the responses that many managers lack the basic techniques and management skills to manage these tricky situations.

Funding cuts continue to affect the whole of the public sector following the economic downturn in 2009–2011 and have resulted in a number of organisations trying to deliver the same level of service with a much-reduced workforce. The recent government mantra for the public sector of doing 'more with less' is guaranteed to cause problems with workplace stress, staff sickness absence and a general reduction in service, and yet so many organisations seem to think that simply loading more and more work onto a diminishing staff base will have no effect.

The situation in some FRSs is exacerbated by the fact that brigade managers have little or no idea how many hours are being worked by their uniformed staff; the findings clearly showed that a large number of employees routinely work more hours than their contacts stipulated for a wide variety of reasons. While it is of course up to individuals to decide whether to donate their own time to their employers, it makes it very hard for an organisation to fully assess its strength when it is making redundancy decisions. Whether a decision to work longer hours is a personal one, or one encouraged by a manager or simply dictated by circumstances, the findings show that there is an implicit expectation that staff will put in many extra hours. And the danger here is also that tired people make poor decisions, and firefighters work in a safety critical environment.

A related problem for the employers is that of presenteeism: when staff come into work even though they are unwell, or simply stay longer at work in order to be noticed and considered to be loyal. Several respondents reported working regularly more hours than they were contracted to, and yet there was no evidence that the organisation was more productive as a result. Indeed, evidence was mentioned in the literature review to suggest that presenteeism actually reduces productivity regardless of the reason why employees are putting in their extra hours. This practice should be discouraged as it does little for the overall productivity and effectiveness of the organisation. A further aspect of this presenteeism is the tendency of firefighters to not take all of their earned rota days, holidays and time off in lieu. If a flexi-duty officer works on 24-h cover over a weekend and then fails to take their allotted rota days, the net result is that the officer could be working 12 consecutive days without a break, and the quality of their decision-making must surely be suspect. A very salutary lesson can be gained by reading the US Chemical Safety and Hazard Investigation Board report (2007) on the BP oil refinery explosion in March 2005 at Texas City (which killed 15 people and injured 180). The report points to a combination of relentless cost-cutting, inadequate monitoring and supervision, and the increased levels of overwork and fatigue of the operational staff. There are many other examples that illustrate the fact that simply expecting the remaining staff members to take on the additional workloads of their former colleagues will not result in currently high-quality work being continued.

The most straightforward way to eliminate the risks of burnout, fatigue and cognitive weariness is to reassess and improve job design and job resources in order to reduce job demands to a manageable level. To design or redesign the job in order to improve the job resources at a time of economic constraint may seem to be a daunting task, but good job resources such as improved internal communications; supportive managers, supervisors and team members; support from HR for managers when taking difficult decisions are not impossible to achieve, nor are they an expensive option, and yet they could create significant improvements. Whereas poor job resources such as irregular and complex shift patterns, uncaring and ineffective managers, low levels of peer support (often combined with high levels of competition for a relatively few choice positions) and potentially hazardous working conditions are bound to create a situation where high levels of stress, fatigue, burnout and cognitive weariness are more likely (Mostert 2011). Such basic improvements are likely to have an additional benefit: that of improved work-home interface, so that there should be fewer problems from home life leeching into the work arena. Despite the fact that managers did not understand that situations at home can influence the health and wellbeing of their team members, they did seem to understand that improving those situations for themselves will have a beneficial effect, and so job design is an important tool in retaining and enhancing the skills and motivation of the workforce. It is well known that motivated workers are more productive, healthy workers have fewer days off sick and workers who feel appreciated will continue to offer their skills to the organisation.

The impact of shift working on the wellbeing and management of older firefighters presents a challenge to any organisation required to provide a service at all times of the day or night. While there has been a steady decrease in the number of domestic house fires, the FRS still has to be available to respond quickly to a wide range

of other non-fire-related emergency incidents such as flooding, road traffic collisions and even the threat of terrorism. So shift working is bound to continue. The
challenge is how to maintain an efficient emergency service while accommodating
the health and wellbeing (and therefore the productivity) of the ageing workforce.
The physical demands of the job are sometimes more difficult to cope with, and
older workers may require extra time to get over injuries and complex shift patterns.
However, some respondents preferred working shifts as it gave them the opportunity to spend more time with their family, for example, collecting the children from
school or taking them on days out. Problems for these people had arisen when their
shifts had changed or they had moved from shifts to working Monday to Friday 9–5;
this was a transition point in their family life that many had found an inconvenience.
Often, this change in working conditions had happened at the same time as change
in their personal situation, for example, when an illness or minor injury required
them to request less physical activity.

Although some of the early research on the effects of shift working on older
workers was equivocal (Smith et al. 1998), later authors (e.g. Bohle et al. 2010) have
suggested that older workers take longer to recover from irregular shift patterns
such as those worked by operational firefighters. Skinner et al. (2010) contradict this
by suggesting that the age group most likely to suffer fatigue from long working
hours and irregular shifts are slightly younger at 34–44, although men generally are
more likely to take longer to recover from shift working patterns. Several respondents commented on the increased recovery time needed after night shifts, now they
are getting older and that the lost family time was detrimental to satisfactory family
interactions.

Promotion to a more senior role, whether temporary or substantive, can impact
working hours by placing the manager on the flexi-duty rota. This can in some cases
increase the number of hours that the manager has to be available for work from 42
to 72 each week by being on cover two nights a week and one full weekend in six.
While it is not likely that serious incidents would occur every time the manager is
on cover, they still have to be ready to respond and that can impact family life.
Consideration could be given to the recommendations by Lancashire FRS and others to introduce self-rostering for flexi-duty officers.

Many respondents said that while they had been happy to work shifts when
younger, they were finding it more difficult to recover from the night shifts as they
got older. This comment had been made frequently by those who found that, as they
were getting older, they were experiencing increased tiredness. This could have a
major impact on the Fire and Rescue Service following the abolition of the Default
Retirement Age and the changes to the Firefighters Pension Scheme; uniformed
staff will be expected to continue working beyond the previous retirement age in
order to receive their pension and be able to work beyond State Pension Age. While
those in an administrative or support role might have less difficulty in continuing
their work beyond their expected retirement age, this is likely to be more challenging for older firefighters, whose roles are more physically demanding. One option
could be to offer older firefighters' roles or tasks that are less physical, such as driving appliances; however, the current expectation is that all firefighters should be

competent in all their roles. There are, of course, plenty of roles that do not require the same levels of physical activity, for example, training, HR, administration, and there are sometimes opportunities for firefighters to return to employment in a non-uniformed capacity following retirement, so it should be possible to find a way to move staff onto less physically demanding roles if the need arises.

It used to be the case that the majority of older workers in the Fire and Rescue Service were non-uniformed staff, working on Green Book contracts, contributing to local authority pension schemes requiring them to work until 60/65, rising to 66 and beyond for both men and women by December 2020, so older firefighters were quite rare. As the non-uniformed staff already work beyond 60 in order to gain their pension, the question might be asked whether there are any lessons to be learnt regarding management, motivation, efficiency and productivity of the current older workers. The second study into the management of older workers in the FRS would suggest that many younger managers find the management and motivation of their older colleagues to be problematic, which has often led to reluctance to deal effectively with demotivated or unproductive staff; the irony being that the demotivation is often a result of poor management!

This is not the case in every FRS, there is somewhere the management of the older workforce is taken very seriously, with policies being introduced to ensure that extended working lives are healthy and fulfilled. Of the 14 responses to the brief questionnaire, the majority replied that they had no policies designed for their older workers, nor had any intention of introducing any, commenting that all of their policies were available to all staff regardless of age or role. Four FRSs did have extensive policies and programmes to support their older staff and could act as exemplars of excellent practice.

As most of the firefighters questioned were approaching their retirement, it had been assumed that individuals would be planning in terms of not only financial security but also their social activities and any future work activity. What was surprising was that, when first asked about their retirement plans, nearly half of the respondents (48%) said they were not making any plans; although when questioned further, most of them did have some idea of what they intended to do after they retired. While choosing to plan for retirement can be said to be a deliberate decision, usually reaching a conclusion based on research of the available facts, what decision is made about not making plans? Is this a deliberate decision to not plan? Or is it decision to not think about retirement? It could be simple procrastination or even a reluctance to think about the future, and of course, failure to plan for retirement is not confined to the employees of the Fire and Rescue Service and may have more to do with a lack of understanding of what retirement will actually be like (Goodwin and O'Connor 2014).

Looking at the policies that might be put in place to support older firefighters, most of the English Fire and Rescue Services that responded said that they do offer some type of retirement planning, although most only arrange financial advice a few months before retirement – when it is too late to change anything. A few others have introduced extensive pre-retirement programmes that cover all aspects of retirement: *We do hold pre-retirement courses a few years prior to the expected date of retirement to help plan staff for the practical, financial and emotional aspects retirement might present.* There is considerable research to show that good planning and control over the retirement process greatly improves health and wellbeing in the years following retirement (Calvo et al. 2009; Loretto and Vickerstaff 2013).

As the number of female firefighters increases, so too does the number of older female firefighters, and many will experience additional challenges during the menopause, particularly when wearing breathing apparatus. When asked whether there were organisational policies to cover this point, most respondents stated that they were 'waiting for CFOA to devise a policy', but a few include extensive menopause policies within their general Occupational Health (OH) provisions. *We also offer a course to females on Menopause Self Care. This one day intensive course offers support to find ways to: Improve nutrition and make informed lifestyle choices, To research and review your own requirements, To voice your feelings and concerns more clearly.*

For general health and fitness issues, most FRSs state they were using their Occupational Health departments to encourage improved fitness, particularly among midlife and older firefighters:

> *We have a fitness at work policy which provides for all ages of staff and is non-discriminatory in terms of age. This assesses firefighters health and fitness to do all tasks – it does not make specific issue of 'menopausal' firefighter's but we do provide a full occupational health service with information provision specific to a number of age related conditions and physiological deteriorations - including eyesight, hearing etc. In terms of wearing of breathing apparatus and menopause specifically, we are aware of the issues of core temperature fluctuation but do not have a specific policy on it. We do however employ Equivital core monitoring for FBT training and also undertake ear temperature monitoring prior to controlled hot wear exposures, though this is obviously impractical at incidents.*

Even in those Fire and Rescue Services that do not have a specific policy, there was anecdotal evidence that crews and watches made their own arrangements to accommodate the needs of menopausal women in breathing apparatus, although ad hoc arrangements do not provide an answer for the national FRS.

A substantial proportion of older firefighters will have to care for sick or elderly relatives in addition to their paid employment. However, very few FRSs have any specific policies, relying instead upon the 'we treat everyone the same' mantra, possibly in the mistaken belief that age-related policies are somehow contrary to the age discrimination legislation (Parry and Tyson 2011).

Considering this from an Occupational Health perspective, the FRS will have to make provision for a much larger cohort of older firefighters than before; for example, are they still fit enough to undertake the full range of operational duties? If not, will they be allocated less physical roles, which in turn could impact the competence of other firefighters? Are there enough semi-operational roles for the older workers, for example, full fitness is probably not required to go into schools and community groups to talk about fire safety or to fit smoke alarms. A distinct advantage of having more older operational staff is that vital skills, knowledge and experience can be retained within the organisation, and older firefighters can mentor and guide younger members of staff on a more structured basis than currently obtained.

Managing and motivating older firefighters is something that many managers find difficult, often as they have all been part of the same team for many years. But instead of spending time seeking answers to problems, many managers use performance management or capability to manage older firefighters out of the service as a quick short-term solution. This has the effect of denying the FRS of years of experience, expertise, knowledge and skill and leaving the FRS with considerable skills gaps. This is sometimes remedied by re-engaging their 'retirees' as consultants or non-uniformed staff, which is often more expensive. A more effective way of transferring that knowledge would be to have a formal mentoring scheme so that older firefighters could pass their knowledge and experience on to their younger colleagues. Many organisations have a cross-mentoring programme where younger workers assist their older colleagues with new technology and work practices.

Recommendations

If firefighters are going to work for 40 years before qualifying for their pensions, how should the FRS manage the health, wellbeing, motivation and productivity of its older workforce, while ensuring the safety of other employees as well as the community at large?

Firstly, they must concentrate on management training that acknowledges the value of the older firefighter rather than seeing them as a problem. Good management of the entire organisation should result in all firefighters (including older firefighters) feeling valued, well trained and fit enough to do the work. Tasnim's call *To create a healthy and happy workplace, the organization must focus on developing a positive psychology, self-esteem, job engagement, job satisfaction, safety at workplace, freedom, valued social position, stress management and work-family conciliation (Tasnim 2016)* should not be seen as economically impossible or inconvenient, but one that makes sound common sense, improving managers' 'cross-generational' management skills, so that they communicate more effectively with different age groups. Motivation and performance management are skills that can be easily taught. There is considerable evidence that so-called age-related decline has little to do with chronological age and much more to do with peer interaction and issues of selection for training (Myck 2015).

From an Occupational Health perspective, fire services should consider redesigning and reassigning some job roles where fitness is a factor. Where physical fitness is a requirement, then it behoves the organisation to encourage continued fitness throughout a working life and particularly for those firefighters who take on more sedentary roles as they progress through the organisation's management structure.

Services should use all the skills, qualifications and experience of your older firefighters (after all, you have paid for it!). Encourage mentoring and buddying with younger firefighters to exchange knowledge and experience. This is most effective when two-way or peer mentoring is adopted. Resist the temptation to treat your ageing workforce as a problem; they are a valuable resource, just waiting to be asked for help, advice and commitment, so use it.

Finally, enable and encourage older firefighters to plan properly for all aspects of their retirement: mid-career planning, pre-retirement courses, financial wellbeing checks, health and fitness check-ups should all become the norm. It is not at all helpful to wait until 6 months before someone leaves, as they have no time to make the appropriate changes to their finances or their lifestyle.

References

Beers, H., & Butler, H. (2012). *Age related changes and safety critical work: Identification of tools and a review of the literature.* Health & Safety Laboratory HSE.

Bohle, P., Pitts, C., & Quinlan, M. (2010). Time to call it quits? The safety and health of older workers. *Workplace Health and Quality of Life: International Surveys International Journal of Health Services, 40*(1), 23–41.

Calvo, E., Haverstick, K., & Sass, S. A. (2009). Gradual retirement, sense of control, and retirees' happiness. *Research on Aging, 31*(1), 112–135.

Department for Communities and Local Government. (2008). *Working in the fire service: A survey of current and ex-firefighters in England.* Fire Research Technical Report 8/2008 HMSO.

Department for Communities and Local Government. (2012). *Fire and rescue operational statistics bulletin for England 2011–12.* HMSO.

Farrow, A., & Reynolds, F. (2012). Health and safety of the older worker. *Occupational Medicine, 62*(1), 4–11.

Frankel, L. P., & Picascia, S. (2008). Workplace legacy: Making the most of the final five. *Employment Relations Today Spring, 35*(1), 1–7, Wiley.

Goodwin, J., & O'CONNOR, H. (2014). Notions of fantasy and reality in the adjustment to retirement. *Ageing & Society, 34*(4), 569–589.

Hassell, B. L., & Perrewe, P. L. (1995). An examination of beliefs about older workers: Do stereotypes still exist? *Journal of Organizational Behaviour, 16*, 457–468.

Hutchison, E. D. (2010). *Dimensions of Human behaviour: The changing life course* (4th ed.). Thousand Oaks: Sage.

Joe, C., Patel, K., & Yoong, P. (2013). Knowledge loss when older experts leave knowledge-intensive organisations. *Journal of Knowledge Management, 17*, 6.

Kelloway, K., & Barling, J. (2010). Leadership development as an intervention in occupational health psychology. *Work & Stress: An International Journal of Work, Health & Organisations, 24*, 3.

Loretto, W., & Vickerstaff, S. (2013). The domestic and gendered context for retirement. *Human relations, 66*(1), 65–86.

Moen, P., Erickson, W. A., Agarwal, M., Fields, V., & Todd, L. (2000). *The Cornell retirement and well-being study.* Ithaca, NY: Bronfenbrenner Life Course Center, Cornell University.

Mostert, K. (2011). Job characteristics, work–home interference and burnout: Testing a structural model in the south African context. *The International Journal of Human Resource Management, 22*(5), 1036–1053. March 2011.

Myck, M. (2015). Living longer, working longer: The need for a comprehensive approach to labour market reform in response to demographic changes. *International Journal of Ageing, 12*(1), 3–5.

Parry, E., & Tyson, S. (2011). *Managing an age diverse workforce.* Basingstoke/New York: Palgrave Macmillan.

Pritchard, K., & Whiting, R. (2014). Baby boomers and the lost generation: On the discursive construction of generations at work. *Organization Studies, 35*(11), 1605–1626.

Rego, A., Vitória, A., Cunha, M. P. E., Tupinambá, A., & Leal, S. (2016, Feb). Developing and validating an instrument for measuring managers' attitudes toward older workers. *The International Journal of Human Resource Management, 2016*, 1–34.

Skinner, N., Parvazian, S., & Dorrian, J. (2010). *FLAWS in our lives: Fatigue, work and life strain.* Adelaide: Centre for Work + Life, University of South Australia.

Smith, L., Folkard, S., Tucker, P., & Macdonald, I. (1998). Work shift duration: A review comparing eight hour and 12 hour shift systems. *Occupational Environmental Medicine, 55*, 217–229.

Tasnim, Z. (2016). Happiness at workplace: Building a conceptual framework. *World Journal of Social Sciences, 6*(2), 62–70. July 2016 Special Issue.

US Chemical Safety and Hazard Investigation Board. (2007). *Investigation report: Refinery explosion and fire (15 Killed, 180 injured) BP Texas City 23rd March 2005.* Report No 2005-04-I-TX March 2007.

Dr. Anita Pickerden   runs a coaching and training business specialising in work-life balance and older workers. She is also an Associate Lecturer at Worcester Business School, providing work-based learning programmes. Her doctoral research was on 'the work life balance of older workers in the Fire & Rescue Service as they approach and transition through retirement', and this has led to the design and delivery of training and coaching of both older workers and their younger managers. She continues to research and write about the ways in which organisations manage their ageing workforce.

Chapter 10
Feeling the Heat? Management Reform and Workforce Diversity in the English Fire Service

Rhys Andrews and Rachel Ashworth

Introduction

As discussed in Chaps. 1 and 2, the Labour government in the UK made a concerted effort to modernise the way in which fire brigades are managed and staffed (see Fitzgerald 2005). Modernisation involved the introduction of new duties around fire prevention, reformed pay structures, an integrated development programme for fire service personnel and a renewed emphasis on positive working conditions. An important plank of this agenda for change was an emphasis on management reform designed to increase gender and minority ethnic representation amongst fire brigade staff (Office of the Deputy Prime Minster (ODPM 2003a). The drive to modernise the fire service workforce in part mirrored similar efforts across public services in the UK (Andrews and Ashworth 2013, 2015; Loveday 2006; Colgan et al. 2009). The emphasis on recruiting a more diverse workforce has been further reinforced by the growth in legislation governing the public sector workplace. A new set of equality duties aimed to shift the burden of responsibility from the individual to the public organisation and, to a degree, takes organisations beyond notions of administrative justice (Newman and Ashworth 2016) and overlays the business case for equality with concerns of social justice (Dickens 2006). Previous attempts at reforming the fire service proved difficult, largely due to the nature of the work-based culture that has long characterised the service (Ward and Winstanley 2006). However, this change was compounded by the wider context of public service modernisation and the duty placed on English local authorities (including fire brigades) to promote equality and diversity (ODPM 2001). Consequently, fire service progress against diversity and other targets associated with the modernisation agenda was verified and assessed by the then Audit Commission through its programme of Comprehensive

R. Andrews • R. Ashworth (✉)
Cardiff Business School, Cardiff University, Cardiff, UK
e-mail: ashworthre@cardiff.ac.uk

© Springer International Publishing AG 2018

P. Murphy, K. Greenhalgh (eds.), *Fire and Rescue Services*,
DOI 10.1007/978-3-319-62155-5_10

Performance Assessments (CPA) and the collection and analysis of Best Value Performance Indicator (BVPI) data.

The aim of this chapter is to establish whether management reforms in English fire brigades influenced levels of gender and minority ethnic representation in those organisations. In the first part of this chapter, we begin by discussing how the distinctiveness of fire-fighting as an occupation has posed a challenge to the introduction of management reforms. We then highlight the links between the introduction of new management practices and improvements in the representation of women and minority ethnic groups within organisation. Thereafter, we describe the details of the management reforms introduced in the English fire service. Following that, we describe our data and the methods used to evaluate the relationship between management reform and variations in workforce diversity. Finally, we present and interpret our results before discussing the implications of our findings.

Fire-Fighting as an Occupation

Government efforts to reform the management of the UK fire service have traditionally been met with a considerable degree of (union-led) resistance. It is argued that this opposition to change has primarily been due to the deeply embedded occupational culture within the service that has been evidenced through, the surprisingly few, studies of fire-fighters. Three elements tend to combine to shape this culture: high levels of workplace trade unionism (still more than 80%); the close-knit and 'dirty' nature of the occupation; and homogeneity within the workforce.

In their review of attempts at organisational restructuring in the fire service in the 1990s, Fitzgerald and Stirling (1999: 58) describe the culture of workplace trade unionism and argue that it is essential to understanding failures to reform the service:

> the action of the FBU (Fire Brigades Union) can be characterised by a resilient, conservative, defensive, militancy built on a culture of collectivism that supports trade unionism and is resistant to changes that challenge either service provision or conditions of service.

It is argued that the trade union culture not only shapes the behaviour of fire-fighters, but also those who become managers within the service, as a result of their collective working experiences within the watch system (Fitzgerald 2005). Within the context of diversity, at a national level, the Fire Brigades Union (FBU) has actively promoted equality and fairness in the workplace for over 20 years. The policy document 'All Different, All Equal' (FBU 2007) provides a recent example of the emphasis given at national level to outlawing discrimination and reinforcing a culture of dignity and respect across the service. However, although he states the service has 'come a long way', the then President Mick Shaw also acknowledged that 'we still have members whose working lives are being made intolerable due to the unacceptable behaviour of their colleagues' (2007:3).

The intense debate about the role of trade unions in promoting and ensuring the implementation of equal opportunities policies suggests that the national and local

FBU responses to equality reform are likely to be especially important. It is hoped that unions will play out a leadership role in relation to equality but early research into the existence and substance of equal opportunities policies questions this assumption. For example, Hoque and Noon reported in 2004 that unionised workplaces are more likely to have equal opportunities policies but that these tended to be 'empty shells' (497). Some attribute this partly to a failure of capacity as union density declines whilst others have pointed to a failure of will (Heery 2010). It has been argued that the need to protect membership interests results in union policy at the local level which has negative consequences for equality. For example, Jenkins et al. (2002) observed a wide variation in local union practices with the consequence that, in some cases, unions engage in restricting opportunities for over-time to full-time workers, thereby excluding part-time (mostly female workers). They go onto conclude that 'such practices seriously question the ability of some trade unions to deliver equality in the workplace' (101).

Others are more optimistic and whilst they acknowledge the ways in which unions have undermined equalities in the workplace, they document a changing approach, which they attribute to a changing membership and the role of union equality officers (Kirton and Greene 2006). Further, recent analysis of UK WERS data by Bacon and Hoque (2010) reveals that the range of equality and diversity practices has widened within union-recognised workforces, leading them to speculate that 'unions may well be having a significant influence on the EO practices adopted by British employers' (17), although it should be noted that they also express concern about low levels of trade union involvement in negotiation over equality policies.

The highly unionised nature of the fire service is particularly significant when considered alongside the strength of the service's occupational culture. Strong occupational cultures tend to develop when the membership of a group has been stable over time and when members share experiences which then become reinforced by rituals, symbols and routines (Langfield-Smith 1992). These conditions are evident within the fire service. For example, teamwork has been of major importance within the context of the workplace where fire-fighters have traditionally been required not only to work together but also to eat, socialise and sleep as a group (Hall et al. 2007). This close-knit way of working within small units – or 'watches' – has combined with an emphasis on discipline, rank and power to form a culture which has been described as verging on the 'paramilitary' (Archer 1999) with fire-fighting being likened to 'going to war', leading to the frequent inclusion of fire-fighting within categories of uniformed/armed services employment (Yarnal et al. 2004). Fire-fighting has been described as 'dirty work' where tasks vary from the highly dangerous to the most unpleasant. Despite the fact that fire-fighters are admired by the public, enjoy considerable prestige and status and fire-fighting is 'considered to be a masculine form of heroism' (Yarnal et al. 2004), Tracy and Scott (2006) refer to the occupation as one which is 'rife with taint' and report in their research that fire-fighters prioritise and publicise the valorous (and dangerous) aspects of their work (e.g. entering burning buildings) and de-emphasise the more mundane and unpleasant aspects, such as dealing with homeless people and drug addicts. The nature of the fire service culture is clearly shaped by the type of work undertaken by fire-fighters, the close proximity in which they work and live and a traditional emphasis on discipline and authority.

The fire service workplace culture has been further reinforced by a workforce that constitutes a homogenous set of employees who are predominantly white and male (Archer 1999; Yarnal et al. 2004). Some argue that the lack of diversity has been sustained by the workplace culture – 'that is not to say women are unsuited to the job but that the occupation and its culture have been created in a way that sets up barriers to females' (Moore and Kleiner 2001: 209). The service has also been subject to persistent accusations of discrimination and harassment – for example, a study of equal opportunities in the mid-1990s revealed that many women and minority ethnic fire-fighters had suffered from verbal hostility and, on some occasions, harassment and physical abuse (Bucke 1994: 7). Similarly, Yoder and Aniakudo (1995) report that African American female fire-fighters suffer frequent forms of harassment such as 'teasing, jokes and remarks – forms of gender harassment indicative of a hostile work environment' (267). They define the harassment in this case, not solely in terms of the behaviour of fire-fighters but in terms of 'the climate or culture in which it occurs'.

Bucke (1994) reports that, in comparison with the armed forces, police and healthcare, the UK fire service is viewed by potential minority and female applicants as providing low levels of equality and seen as an unsuitable occupation for women on the grounds of potential sexism. These findings are supported by more recent analyses of which demonstrate that the recruitment of women into the service has prompted a negative reaction, mostly in relation to the potential disruption to norms, ways of working and social practices (see, e.g. Hall et al. 2007). Often women recruits are siloed into particular roles or assignments, such as that of the fire-fighter paramedic, highlighting that potentially women may be subject to 'glass walls' in addition to the usual 'glass ceiling' (Hulett et al. 2008).

Overall, the fire service has been characterised by high levels of unionisation, dirty but valorous work and a homogenous set of employees. As Moore and Kleiner (2001: 208) summarise:

> Fire fighting has long been like a fraternity. It has its own special culture like no other job. Fire-fighters live together and often see more of each other than of their own families. The culture is derived from the long history of the fire service, the twenty-four hour shifts, the intense nature of the work and a special camaraderie amongst co-workers. Physical strength, skill and composure are necessary skills for fire-fighters.

The subsequent section of this chapter documents the recent equality and management reforms introduced to the fire service by the UK Government.

Fire Service Reform

Equality Reforms

Fire and rescue authorities have had to collect data on the diversity of their workforce since the establishment of the Best Value programme for improvement in local government. These data reveal that women were underrepresented in the fire service for some time, for example, comprising on average only 12.7% of the workforce of each fire brigade between 2001 and 2006, when they underwent significant reform (and still representing only 14.4% of the workforce in 2014). At the same time, minority ethnic representation was particularly poor, with an average just 1.3% of each fire brigade's workforce coming from a minority ethnic background between 2001 and 2006 (albeit this proportion rose to 4.4% in 2014). The issue of equality and diversity was highlighted within the Bain Report (2002) on the future of the fire service (as discussed in Chaps. 1 and 2) which contained reports of bullying and harassment and suggested that 'the culture of the service has not moved with the times' (p.67). The report recommended that brigades work harder to bring about real improvements and focus on delivering on government targets of 15% female and 9% minority ethnic employees by 2009, though it was emphasised that the focus should be on making change to improve the effectiveness of the service, rather than simply to meet targets.

The service was then placed under sustained pressure from the Labour Government which invested considerably in improving equality and diversity within the fire-fighting workforce. For example, the then Office for the Deputy Prime Minister provided £5 m to support the service in England in implementing a 10-year Equality and Diversity Strategy (2009). That strategy set out a vision for the service (11):

a service that could demonstrate that it serves all communities equally and to the highest standards, building on a closer and more effective relationship with the public and creating a more diverse workforce which better reflects the diversity of the working population in each area.

The Equality and Diversity strategy also marked the extension of existing targets, along with the introduction of new, specific and challenging future targets, designed to help the service to work towards achieving the espoused vision. The ambitious targets suggested that, by 2013, fire authorities should be able to ensure that a minimum of 15% of new entrants to the operational side of the service be women, that they recruit minority staff in line with local populations, and also ensure parity in rates of retention between minority ethnic and white and men and women staff – all targets that have yet to be achieved. In pursuit of the targets, the Equality and Diversity strategy specified action in wider areas of managerial responsibility such as leadership, accountability, service delivery, employment practice, and evaluation and dissemination of good practice. This led to some developments at the national level, such as the Equality and Diversity Awards Programme which rewards and publicises examples of good practice and the introduction of a five-point equality charter for Fire Brigade members. The responsibility for delivering on national actions rested with a range of organisations which include DCLG, the Local Government Association, the Chief Fire Officers' Association and the FBU. In contrast, at the local level, fire brigades were to take prime responsibility for delivering improvement by reviewing their procedures for collecting and analysing staff exit information in order to tackle retention issues, and demonstrating how they are promoting equality and how effective their equality schemes and action plans have been (Fire and Rescue Service 2009).

Management Reform

As stated earlier, the emphasis on equality and diversity coincided with reforms to fire service management, work and organisation. As discussed in Chap. 2, the publication of the Bain Report (2002) marked a watershed for the fire service. Stating that the fire service had fallen behind other areas of the public sector, due to unsatisfactory industrial relations, weak management systems and a lack of ownership by those involved in the service, Bain (2002) advocated that service be reformed 'from top to bottom' (p. ii). Consequently, it was recommended that the fire service be re-oriented towards risk management, community fire safety and fire prevention. These changes were by greater powers for local authorities in relation to employment conditions and the proposed introduction of a new Integrated Personal Development System (IPDS) linked to a significant pay award. The Integrated Personal Development System (IPDS) aimed to reduce the ambiguity around the role of both whole-time and retained (part-time) fire-fighters and was introduced as a requirement on fire brigades as part of the pay agreement in 2003. As a comprehensive role management system, IPDS covers all fire service staff (fire-fighters, control operators and managers) at every stage in their professional development, from entry to retirement. By linking roles to National Occupational Standards, it is intended to enable role holders to attain and maintain established levels of competence through targeted training and development. Allied to the repeal of the pre-existing appointments and promotions regulations for operational staff, it permits recruitment at all levels of the service and links career progression to ability rather than rank and hierarchical position (ODPM 2002).

These management changes were intended to reduce harmful effects of role ambiguity amongst middle managers and front-line staff (Moynihan and Pandey 2007) and promote the benefits of well-designed HRM policies, for example in terms of reducing turnover (Guest et al. 2003). A more managerial approach to running fire services was designed to facilitate 'a new preventative, community-focused and resource-conscious way of working' (McGurk 2009: 468). In this way, the change was deemed important as fire-fighters in England became expected to fulfil new roles associated with the promotion of fire safety, such as providing advice and guidance to local businesses, during the study period (Office of the Deputy Prime Minister 2003b). However, the fire service management reforms in the context of diversity were especially important for two reasons. Firstly, as stated above, the changes in recruitment policy may result in an increasing emphasis being placed upon ability, rather than rank or position, which should help to ensure that recruitment and selection processes are fairer and more open. Secondly, the changes strengthen the strategic importance of the HR function within the fire service. Equal opportunities policies can be more meaningful and less of an 'empty shell' when this scenario occurs – see, for example, the work of Hoque and Noon (2004) which demonstrates that HR specialists fulfil a 'guardian role'. However, as Woodhams and Lupton (2006) point out, the lack of status amongst HR officers can encourage negotiation and compromise between HR and line managers, which potentially leads to breaches of equality policies (80).

Although fire brigades have yet to meet the ambitious targets originally laid out in the Equality and Diversity strategy, the operational statistics highlight that the fire service has become a little more representative of the female and minority ethnic populations that they served during the past 10–15 years (see https://www.gov.uk/government/collections/fire-and-rescue-authorities-operational-statistics). Nevertheless, it is important at this stage to examine the data on the fire service workforce for 2001–2006 in order to determine whether the management reforms introduced by the Labour government at that time actually made any difference. The next section of this chapter describes the methodology employed and presents an analysis of the picture across the fire service in England during the reform period.

Data and Methodology

The data set presented in this chapter covers all 46 English fire brigades between the years 2002 and 2006. Each of these fire brigades were governed by elected representatives appointed by the major local authorities within the geographical area that they serve. Brigades were responsible for setting the budget and determining service delivery arrangements for a wide range of fire and rescue services within their jurisdiction, including fire suppression and prevention, accident response and emergency resilience. Our evaluation of workforce diversity in English fire brigades focuses on the representation of women and minority ethnic groups. Although the Labour government's Equality and Diversity strategy covered other equality strands, such as disability, data on these characteristics were not available for the study period.

Workforce Diversity

The data used to measure workforce diversity are drawn from a set of Best Value Performance Indicators (BVPIs) published by the Audit Commission for the study period. These indicators were collected by the Audit Commission as important indicators of 'corporate health' and were intended to give a snapshot of the 'underlying capacity and performance' of local authorities (Department for Environment, Transport and the Regions 2000: 12). The specific measures of diversity we draw upon include the BVPI measuring the percentage of the total workforce that is from minority ethnic groups, and two BVPIs measuring 'the percentage of the top 5% of earners that are women' and 'the percentage of the top 5% of earners that are of minority ethnic origin'. In addition, supplement the BVPI data with data on the percentage of the total workforce that is female drawn from the fire service operational statistics published annually by the Department for Communities and Local Government (www.communities.gov.uk/fire/researchandstatistics/firestatistics/firerescue/).

Determinants of Diversity

The key independent variables measuring management reform and other relevant organisational and environmental factors that we include in our explanatory model are detailed next. Each of them was collected for the year prior to the dependent variables to ensure that causality runs in the expected direction.

Management Reform

Measures of management reform are available for the first 2 years of its implementation. To monitor the introduction of the IPDS and other systems, central government introduced a verification procedure classifying fire brigades on 'how successfully they are modernising' using a traffic light system (green – good progress, amber – some progress, red – little or no progress) (Audit Commission 2004). This modernisation verification programme was then superseded by CPA in 2005 which graded each fire brigade's performance on a four-point scale of 'Inadequate', 'Adequate', 'Performing well' and 'Performing strongly'. Fire brigades' scores on modernisation were therefore taken as measures of the impact of management reform.

Organisation size Conventional economic arguments suggest that larger organisations can spread fixed central costs (e.g. senior management team, information technology, premises) across a wider range and higher quantity of service outputs (Stigler 1958), thereby permitting the release of more resources for the organisational development. Big fire brigades may also be able to increase levels of professional specialisation and expertise, and attract better-quality staff and politicians (Davies 1969). Furthermore, research shows that more proactive equality policies are associated with larger workplaces (Andrews and Ashworth 2013). Data on the total number of employees in each fire brigade for 2001–2005 are therefore used to assess the potential influence of scale economies on workforce diversity.

Fire Brigade Expenditure Equality and diversity legislation requires that fire brigades promote workforce diversity within the organisation. To do so effectively, brigades may need to devote considerable additional resources to new approaches to recruitment, retention, development programmes and other human resource issues over and above their usual service operating and back office costs. Fire brigade expenditure per capita between 2001 and 2005 is therefore taken as a measure of total resources expended by each organisation.

Unionisation A proxy for the relative influence of unionisation on fire service workforce issues was included in the multivariate models: the percentage of seats on the fire brigade governing board held by the Labour Party. In the absence of detailed comprehensive data on levels of FBU membership within fire brigades, the measure is a useful proxy for the potential effects of unionisation. The relationship between Labour support and membership FBU is in part likely to reflect the association

Table 10.1 Descriptive statistics for independent variables

	Mean	Min	Max	SD
IPDS implementation	2.5	1.0	3.0	.6
Service expenditure per capita	34.2	21.7	61.0	6.9
Population	1082923.4	132,731	7,518,000	1069630.6
% Labour council seats	37.3	2.5	78.4	18.8
Minority ethnic population	4.4	.0	29.0	5.0

between support for Left-wing parties and trade union membership observed across the globe (Riley 1997). At the same time, the FBU and Labour representatives on fire authorities have traditionally enjoyed an especially close working relationship (Fitzgerald 2005). We therefore expect to capture at least some of the effects of unionisation through the use of this measure.

Population diversity It is possible that fire brigades operating in areas with a higher proportion of underrepresented social groups are able to draw upon a larger pool of labour with which to address workforce diversity issues. To assess whether the demographic composition of the areas served by fire brigades influenced levels of minority ethnic representation, we therefore included a measure of the proportion of the population of working age of minority ethnic origin within the models of minority ethnic representation. Since the gender split of the demographic composition of the working population is approximately 50/50, no such measure was used in our models of gender representation. Descriptive statistics for all the variables used in the statistical modelling are shown in Table 10.1.

Findings and Discussion

To explore the patterns of gender and minority ethnic representation in more depth, we carried out multivariate analysis incorporating the management reform scores and our control variables. Table 10.2 presents the results of the panel regression models used to test the impact of these variables on workforce diversity during the study period. Logged versions of population and the proportion of the population of working age of minority ethnic origin were used to correct for skewness. The statistical model is a fixed effects panel regression evaluating the effects of organisational and environmental factors on gender and minority ethnic representation over time within English fire brigades.

The results of our analyses are shown in Table 10.2. Fire service expenditure per capita is statistically significant in the expected direction (positive) in both gender representation models. Although no such result was observed for minority ethnic representation, these findings do point to the possibility that big spending fire brigades devoted more resources to gender equality issues. No such effects are observed for population in any of the models, suggesting organisational size did not matter.

Table 10.2 Determinants of workforce diversity in English fire brigades 2002–2006

	Gender representation				Minority ethnic representation			
	% of total workforce		% of top 5% earners		% of total workforce (log)		% of top 5% earners (log)	
	Slope	z-score	Slope	z-score	Slope	z-score	Slope	z-score
Constant	−133.601	−1.00	519.624	.92	11.220	1.46	17.315	.66
IPDS	.271	2.25*	−.007	−.01	.016	2.21*	.052	2.19*
Expenditure per capita	.121	4.18**	.429	3.56**	.001	.78	−.005	−.90
Population (log)	23.927	1.06	−89.480	−.94	−1.847	−1.42	−2.882	−.65
% Labour council seats	−.007	−.57	.025	.49	−.001	−1.55	.001	.42
Minority ethnic working population (log)					.054	1.13	.022	.13
F-statistic	27.23**		3.44**		7.01**		.95	
Within R^2	.52		.12		.24		.04	
No. of observations	229		226		229		226	

Note: Significance levels: $*p \leq 0.05$; $**p \leq 0.01$ (two-tailed test)

The coefficient for Labour seats measure is unrelated to gender or minority ethnic representation. Surprisingly, the coefficient for the percentage of the working population of minority ethnic origin, though positive, was not statistically significant. This implies that fire brigades serving large ethnic minority populations seemed to find it as difficult to address issues of race equality as their counterparts in less ethnically diverse areas. Table 10.2 shows that the coefficient for management reform is positive and statistically significant in three out of the four models, indicating that better implementation of systems such as IPDS is associated with improvements on workforce diversity. It is possible that IPDS strengthened the HR function within the fire service and that management reform triggered changes in the recruitment behaviour of fire brigades and made the service more attractive to potential applicants. These data therefore suggest that implementing modernisation reforms can have a positive impact on the equality agenda. Indeed, data from the fire and rescue operational statistics for the past 15 years highlight that the rate of improvement in women and ethnic minorities' representation in the workforce of fire brigades was greater between 2002 and 2006 than in the following 8 years.

Despite the apparent success of management reform in enhancing representation, it is nevertheless noticeable that its positive effect is more apparent for the diversity of the workforce as a whole, than in the upper echelons. Whilst the coefficient is positive and statistically significant in the model of minority ethnic representativeness in top management, it is important to note that this model as whole does not furnish a statistically significant explanation of the variations in the rate of top 5% earners being of minority ethnic origin (the f-statistic is below 1). It is clear that the fire service faces issues of uneven representation at multiple levels of its organisation and consequently strategies for improving patterns of diversity should vary accordingly. It may be that these data reflect the results of increased activity aimed at attracting new recruits to lower levels of the organisation. However, efforts at improving the very poor levels of representation at the upper echelons of the service require attention not only to recruitment but also to ensuring fair systems of progression and promotion. Whilst some suggest that the growing presence of female staff within the fire service may lead to 'shifting understandings' of the occupational requirements for fire-fighting (Hall et al. 2007), Agocs and Burr (1996) remind us that policies, such as those aimed at improving diversity in the fire service through 'numerical representation', do not necessarily result in 'changing organizational practices and climate in order to ensure that, once hired, members of the designated groups would be full and equal participants in the workplace, enjoying equitable career development opportunities and rewards for their contributions' (32). Clearly, extensive qualitative research is required to explore these issues in more depth within the fire service.

Conclusions

This chapter has examined changes in the workforce composition of English fire brigades between 2002 and 2006 in order to evaluate whether the implementation of management reforms influenced patterns of gender and minority ethnic representation. The evidence suggests that there have been some small improvements in the overall diversity of the English fire service workforce and that these may, in part, be attributable to the implementation of management reforms. In particular, overall levels of gender and minority ethnic representation within the workforce of fire brigades seem to have been enhanced by the introduction of certain HR systems. However, representativeness within the upper managerial echelons of these organisations appeared to be untouched by this reform. Given that levels of workforce diversity have not altered much during the past 10 years, changing the composition of the workforce will be a slow process and it will take some considerable time to effect and evidence a more fundamental change within the service. As Archer (1999) points out, the fire-fighting culture has been shaped since the creation of the first fire brigade in 1833 and with female fire-fighters only invited into the service in the last 20 years, slow progress is perhaps inevitable.

Previous research suggests that equality and diversity strategies are difficult to implement in isolation. For example, the new Equality and Diversity Strategy and its associated targets may create a backlash and be met with resistance so, as Newman and Ashworth (2016) argue, it is important that management reforms are underpinned and accompanied by tough change mechanisms, such as new procedures and evaluation tools, along with an attempt to mainstream and embed principles of equality and diversity within the service. There is continued debate over the role that line managers and HR departments play in advancing the equality agenda (McConville 2006), with the role and status of equality officers deemed to be especially crucial, along with high-level organisational championing and support (Conley and Page 2014). There are also a host of organisational factors that are likely to mediate the impact of equality reforms. These have been established previously in relation to the implementation of employment legislation (see, e.g. Dickens and Hall 2006 who point to management style and a predominance of well-informed union members).

Finally, the changing nature of the workforce is just one aspect of the reform programme experienced by the fire service during this time period. There are additional changes associated with modernisation that are likely to impact on the extent and success of diversity reforms. For example, Fitzgerald (2005) argues that reform poses a key challenge to the nature of the occupation as an entirely different skill set is likely to be required for a new fire service, based on prevention. Furthermore, it is possible that management reform dilutes the strength of workplace trade unionism. This chapter reveals a small degree of change within the service but demonstrates the urgent need for further in-depth qualitative research on the impact of management reforms on the diversity of the fire-fighting workforce. It also underlines the value of conducting additional research on the lasting effects of large-scale-managed equality reforms and the role of government policies and regulations in reducing or sustaining inequalities (Ozbligin and Tatli 2011).

References

Agocs, C., & Burr, C. (1996). Employment equity, affirmative action and managing diversity: Assessing the differences. *International Journal of Manpower, 17*(4/5), 30–45.

Andrews, R., & Ashworth, R. (2013). Determinants of representation: An empirical assessment of the UK civil service. *Policy and Politics, 41*(3), 429–448.

Andrews, R., & Ashworth, R. (2015). Representation and inclusion in public organizations: Evidence from the UK civil service. *Public Administration Review, 75*(2), 279–288.

Archer, D. (1999). Exploring "bullying" culture in the para-military organisation. *International Journal of Manpower, 20*(12), 94–105.

Audit Commission. (2004). *Second verification report on the progress of modernisation*. London: Audit Commission.

Bacon, N., & Hoque, K. (2010). Exploring the relationship between union learning representatives and employer-provided training in Britain. *The International Journal of Human Resource Management, 21*(5), 720–741.

Bucke, T. (1994). *Equal opportunities and the fire service*. London: Home Office.

Colgan, F., Wright, T., Creegan, C., & McKearney, A. (2009). Equality and diversity in public services: Moving forward on lesbian, gay and bisexual equality? *Human Resource Management Journal, 19*(3), 280–301.

Conley, H., & Page, M. (2014). *Gender equality in public services: Chasing the dream*. London: Routledge.

Davies, B. (1969). Local authority size: Some associations with standards of performance of services for deprived children and old people. *Public Administration, 47*(2), 225–248.

Department for Environment, Transport and the Regions. (2000). *Best value performance indicators for 2000/2001*. London: HMSO.

Dickens, L. (2006). Re-regulation for gender equality: From 'either/or' to 'both. *Industrial Relations Journal, 37,* 299–309.

Dickens, L., & Hall, M. J. (2006). Fairness – up to a point. Assessing the impact of new labours employment legislation. *Human Resource Management Journal, 16*(4), 338–356.

Fire and Rescue Service. (2009). *Equality and diversity report 2009.* London: FRS.

Fire Brigades Union. (2007). *All different, all equal.* London: FBU.

Fitzgerald, I. (2005). The death of corporatism? Managing change in the fire service. *Personnel Review, 34*(6), 648–662.

Fitzgerald, I., & Sterling, J. (1999). A slow burning flame? Organisational change and industrial relations in the fire service. *Industrial Relations Journal, 30*(1), 46–60.

Guest, D. E., Michie, J., Conway, N., & Sheehan, M. (2003). Human resource management and corporate performance in the UK. *British Journal of Industrial Relations, 41*(2), 291–314.

Hall, A., Hockey, J., & Robinson, V. (2007). Occupational cultures and the embodiment of masculinity: Hairdressing, estate agency and fire fighting. *Gender, Work and Organisation, 14*(6), 534–551.

Heery, E. (2010). Debating employment law: Responses to juridification. In P. Blyton, E. Heery, & P. Turnbull (Eds.), *Reassessing the employment relationship.* London: Palgrave, forthcoming.

Hoque, K., & Noon, M. (2004). Equal opportunities policy and practice in Britain: Evaluating the empty shell hypothesis. *Work, Employment and Society, 18*(3), 481–506.

Hulett, D. M., Bendick, M., Jr., Thomas, S. Y., & Moccio, F. (2008). Enhancing women's inclusion in firefighting in the USA. *International Journal of Diversity in Organisations, Communities & Nations, 8*(2), 189–208.

Jenkins, S., Martinez-Lucio, M., & Noon, M. (2002). Return to gender: An analysis of women's disadvantage in postal work. *Gender, Work and Organization, 9*(1), 81–104.

Kirton, G., & Greene, A. (2006). The discourse of diversity in unionised contexts: Views from trade union equality officers. *Personnel Review, 35*(4), 431–450.

Langfield-Smith, K. (1992). Exploring the need for a shared cognitive map. *Journal of Management Studies, 29*(3), 349–368.

Loveday, B. (2006). Workforce modernisation: Implications for the police service in England and Wales. *The Police Journal, 79*(2), 105–124.

McConville, T. (2006). Devolved HRM responsibilities, middle managers and role dissonance. *Personnel Review, 36*(6), 637–653.

McGurk, P. (2009). Developing 'middle leaders' in the public services? The realities of management and leadership development for public managers. *International Journal of Public Sector Management, 22*(6), 464–477.

Moore, S., & Kleiner, B. H. (2001). Steps to help prevent sexual discrimination from occurring in the fire fighting organisations. *International Journal of Sociology and Social Policy, 21*(8/9/10), 206–218.

Moynihan, D., & Pandey, S. (2007). Finding workable levers over work motivation. *Administration & Society, 39*(7), 803–832.

Newman, J., & Ashworth, R. E. (2016). Changing equalities: Politics, policies and practice. In T. Bovaird & E. Loeffler (Eds.), *Public management and governance* (pp. 297–309). London: Routledge.

ODPM. (2002). *The integrated personal development system,* Fire Service Circular 9/2002.

ODPM. (2003a). *Equality and diversity in local government in England: A literature review.* London: HMSO.

ODPM. (2003b). *Our fire and rescue service.* London: ODPM.

Office for the Deputy Prime Minister (ODPM). (2001). *Strong local leadership – Quality public services.* London: HMSO.

Ozbligin, M., & Tatli, A. (2011). Mapping out the field of equality and diversity: Rise of individualism and voluntarism. *Human Relations, 64*(9), 1229–1253.

Riley, N.-M. (1997). Determinants of union membership: A review. *Labour, 11*(2), 265–301.

Stigler, G. (1958). The economics of scale. *Journal of Law and Economics, 1,* 54–71.

Tracy, S. J., & Scott, C. (2006). Sexuality, masculinity and taint management among fire-fighters and correctional officers: Getting down and dirty with "America's Heroes" and the "scum of law enforcement". *Management Communication Quarterly, 20*(1), 6–38.

Ward, J., & Winstanley, D. (2006). Watching the watch: The UK fire service and its impact on sexual minorities in the workplace. *Gender Work and Organisation, 13*(2), 193–219.

Woodhams, C., & Lupton, B. (2006). Gender-based equal opportunities policy and practice in small firms: The impact of HR professionals. *Human Resource Management Journal, 16*(1), 74–97.

Yarnal, C. M., Dowler, L., & Hutchinson, S. (2004). Don't let the bastards see you sweat: Masculinity, public and private space, and the volunteer firehouse. *Environment and Planning A, 36*(4), 685–699.

Yoder, J. D., & Aniakudo, P. (1995). The responses of African American women firefighters to gender harassment at work. *Sex Roles, 32*(3), 125–137.

Rhys Andrews is Professor of Public Management at Cardiff Business School. He is co-author of Strategic Management and Public Service Performance (2012, Macmillan) and Public Service Efficiency: Reframing the Debate (2014, Routledge), and has published nearly 90 refereed articles in international journals. Rhys is currently co-editor of the Journal of Public Administration Research Theory and the International Public Management Journal, sits on the editorial boards of Public Administration and Local Government Studies, and is an advisor to the Welsh Government's Local Government Finance Distribution Sub-Group and the Data Unit – Wales. His research interests focus on the influence of strategic management and organisational structure on public service outcomes.

Professor Rachel Ashworth is Professor of Public Management at Cardiff Business School. Her research interests include institutional and organisational change in the context of public service reform, public sector accountability and analysing equality, diversity and inclusion in public organisations. Recent research projects have focused on the development of integrated collaborative accountability and the emerging role of Police and Crime Commissioners. Rachel is joint editor of Public Service Improvement: Theories and Evidence (OUP, 2010), is a member of the editorial board of Perspectives on Public Management and Governance and has published in a number of world-leading journals including Journal of Public Administration Research and Theory, Public Administration Review, Public Administration and Journal of Management Studies. She has also provided research evidence to a range of UK government departments and UK Parliament and Welsh Assembly committees.

Chapter 11
The Use of Equality and Equality Frameworks by Fire and Rescue Services

Julian Clarke

Introduction

Fire and Rescue Services (FRSs) came late to improving equality policy and practice in service delivery and employment and to developing risk management processes that allowed them to differentiate between the population categories defined by equality and anti-discrimination legislation. But in the last ten years or so they have made progress; perhaps more than any other set of public service organisations. For example, having had a homophobic reputation in the 1980s and 1990s, things had changed so much that there were two fire appliances with their crews at the Manchester Pride celebrations in August 2016, and Cheshire FRS ranked 13 on Stonewall's Equality Index of its 100 top employers (Stonewall 2016). The importance of equality policy and practice to FRS is well summarised by the Mid-Wales FRS that made the following comments in a recent annual equalities report, enumerating the main business drivers for equality improvement:

- Managing risk and reputation
- Enhancing individual and business performance
- Developing a creative, innovative culture
- Meeting the needs of our communities
- Attracting, retaining and developing employees
- Compliance with legislation

(Mid and West Wales FRS Annual Equality Report 1st April 2012 to 31 March 2013).

This chapter examines the trajectory of equality policy and management practice in fire and rescue services in the UK. The changes in fire service equality

J. Clarke (✉)
Edgehill Business School, Edgehill University, Lancashire, UK
e-mail: clarkej@edgehill.ac.uk

© Springer International Publishing AG 2018   159
P. Murphy, K. Greenhalgh (eds.), *Fire and Rescue Services*,
DOI 10.1007/978-3-319-62155-5_11

policy and practice over the past 20 years have been principally driven by three broadly defined sets of factors:

- A change in emphasis from protection of property to protection of lives brought together by the 2004 Fire Services Act, which centred on the development and maintenance of Integrated Risk Management Plans (IRMP)
- A set of regulatory regimes, awards and comparisons of achievement overseen by the Audit Commission and the Department of Communities and Local Government (DCLG) and reinforced by agencies of the Local Government Association
- Change in equality law and the incorporation of positive action principles, which began with the publication of the Macpherson Report (1999) and included the development of equality performance standards

This chapter takes a historical developmental approach. It starts with a commentary on the concepts of equality and diversity, equal opportunities and equality of outcome. It then briefly explores changes in equality law and the emergence of equality policy and management between 1965 and the Macpherson report of 1999.

The section that follows focuses on the period of major legislative, regulatory and policy development between 2000 and 2010. The introduction of Equality Standard for Local Government (ESLG) and its use by FRS will be discussed and detailed. During engagement with ESLG, FRS produced a range of outputs, particularly a wide range of policy documents relating to both service delivery and employment, to the setting of equality targets in both areas. Eleven out of 47 FRSs sought external assessment of their ESLG achievements.

The last section of this chapter then examines what has happened during the more recent periods of Coalition and Conservative governments after 2010 when ESLG was replaced by a dedicated fire service equality framework subject to peer review and assessment rather than external validation. The detailed regulatory regimes of the previous decade disappeared and were replaced by 'light touch' oversight. It examines whether targets set for positive equality action in service delivery have been followed through by FRS. It examines also equality improvement in employment outcomes, which, for the most part, have been very limited.

Equality and Diversity

In the discussion and formulation of public policy, the concepts of equality and diversity were run together particularly in the 1990s (Ross and Schneider 1992; Kandola et al. 1995). The view taken here is similar to that taken by Rohan Collier in her book on managing equality in service delivery (Collier 1998). It would be impossible to have an equality policy without a diversity component where there is a diverse population to serve and from which to draw staff. But it is quite possible to have a diversity policy without an equality component. Diversity policies may require unequal treatment of certain categories of people; apartheid in South Africa (separate development) was a diversity policy as was segregation in the United States. This is not a trivial point because it is quite possible to have a diverse workforce but one where inequality persists and may be entrenched. An organisation may claim to have a diverse workforce, but if some protected groups (under the 2010 Equality Act) are stuck in its least well-paid staff categories, it may not have an effective equality policy.

The two best known variants of the equality concept are equality of opportunity and equality of outcome. Both concepts and their policy implementations connect in different ways in different contexts (see Arneson 2015). Suffice it to say here that apparent equality of opportunity does not necessarily lead to equality of outcome. In this chapter, equality of outcome will be discussed in relation to both service delivery and employment. Equality in service delivery requires the equal access of a diverse population served by an FRS to the services it provides followed by equal outcomes (in relation to death, injury, and property damage and rescue services). As FRSs have developed their approaches to equality in service delivery, this has meant the assessment of risk to different population categories. One size definitely does not fit all and differential assessment of risk is an essential part of FRS planning. In their approach to employment, we will see that achieving equality of outcome has been difficult in a number of ways although there is well-developed policy and practice that attempts to create equality of opportunity.

For service delivery, equality of opportunity is assessed in terms of equality of outcome (although perhaps not explicitly). If one protected group defined in the terms set out in the 2010 Equality Act is disproportionately adversely affected, then the presumption will be that their opportunity to access services has not been equal in some way. For employment, the situation is more complicated. Certain categories of people are excluded from particular jobs in FRS. So there may appear to be direct disability discrimination in the employment of front-line firefighters but not in employment of non-operational staff. The requirements of the job may create formally legal exceptions. There are, however, examples of firefighters who have returned to work after serious injury and subsequent fitting with prosthetic legs (FBU 2006). 'The physical tests for a front line fire fighter may exclude more women than men from employment but there is notionally no direct discrimination' (UK Fire Resources Group 2014).

Law and Equality Management Before Macpherson

Race, gender and disability equality emerged as public policy issues in different ways between the end of the Second World War and the late 1960s. The Beveridge settlement had defined women and disabled people as (in different ways) being properly supported by the paid labour of able-bodied males (Bagilhole 1997). Women's and disabled people's problems were predominantly seen as welfare issues. Race and ethnicity emerged slowly as a policy issue following non-white

Commonwealth immigration and the introduction of racially targeted immigration control (Miles 1982).

Up to 2000, it is important to note that most equality legislation was framed as anti-discrimination and social cohesion legislation rather than as part of a general policy of civil rights or 'promotion of fair distribution' (Hepple et al. 2000). The three main equality discourses formulated over the past 35 years have been framed in both law and policy outside 'general case' equality politics (what is fair for the whole society) and were directed at ethnic/racial, gender and disability discrimination. They developed within broadly left or socialist perspectives but with interests and demands that are different from and sometimes inconsistent with traditional left politics. The emergence of positive equality duties after 2000 began to change this and began to frame policy that was supposed to positively intervene to lead to a fair or equal distribution of goods and services to various social categories (Neckles 2015).

Race, gender and disability discrimination law emerged unevenly under (primarily) Labour Governments between 1965 and 1995. The problem of racial discrimination/equality emerged out of popular and political reaction to non-white Commonwealth settlement in Britain and subsequent immigration control law (1962 Commonwealth Immigration Act). The 1965 Race Relations Act was initially conceived as a mix of social cohesion and limited anti-discrimination employment law. As race was the first kind of discrimination to be defined as a public policy problem and legislated for, the structure of policy intervention here provided the basic model for all discrimination/equality policy. Housing became a focus with the 1968 Race Relations Act (Daniel 1968).

Local authority and voluntary efforts had focused on integration and welfare in the 1950s and early 1960s. The 1976 Race Relations Act gave local authorities a specific positive duty. The local authority race equality duty, enacted as section 71 of the Race Relations Act 1976, was the first positive Public Sector Equality Duty (PSED) but it only applied to local authorities. It has been argued that the duty demonstrated a government commitment rather than pointing to any specific policy. As a consequence, it had *limited and inadequate guidance and an inadequate regulatory and enforcement framework* (Neckles 2015). The idea of a positive equality duty was, as we will see, reinvigorated more than 20 years later.

Early disability legislation in 1944 and its 1958 successor were pieces of quota or positive discrimination legislation. They were, however, the antithesis of modern equality legislation. They were deemed ineffective in a series of reports (Thornton and Lunt 1993). The Disability Discrimination Act (DDA) (1995) was the first modern anti-disability discrimination statute because disability had been previously seen (in policy terms) as a medical, welfare or special treatment issue: People with impairments were to be helped not given the right to have equal access to jobs and services.

Barbara Bagilhole provided one of the few pieces of detailed local government research done in a large but unnamed county council. Her object of study was Labour controlled and the controlling group set out to use section 71 of the 1976 Race Relations Act to, 'change the under-representation of black and disabled people in the council and the under-representation of women in positions of seniority and power' (Bagilhole 1993, p.163). During the 1980s, council officers had operated with a multiculturalist/assimilationist perspective and did not recognise institutional discrimination as a problem. Their focus was on black communities not on white power structures (Bagilhole 1993). The council established an equal opportunities administrative structure together with a range of consultative mechanisms. The Labour group faced resistance from senior officers who apparently did not feel that councillors had any business modifying policy and committee structures (Bagilhole 1993). Conservative councillors were vocal in opposition and used this in electoral campaigning (Bagilhole 1993). These developments occurred during a period when in certain Labour strongholds a radical equal opportunities approach took hold. There is no evidence that FRS took up any of the equality challenges posed by the 1976 Act.

In 1998, Rohan Collier published a ground breaking book on the management of equality improvement in service delivery (Collier 1998). Heavily influenced by the work of the Commission for Racial Equality (CRE), it outlines all the essential elements of an equality mainstreaming process. It detailed the case for a systematic approach to active management of equality improvement. It showed how service delivery can discriminate both directly and indirectly; what the law required; how different sets of service needs could be identified (one size does not fit all); how policies and action plans could be developed. It indicated the centrality of both performance indicators and effective outcome monitoring and the importance of review and change (equality impact assessment). There is also a chapter on barriers to achieving equality that examined potential resistance from an organisation's staff and from its service users. It is not clear how widely read Collier's book was, but the county council described by Bagilhole and other mainly London metropolitan councils were trying to construct equality improvement programmes that at least paralleled the processes outlined in her book. Larger London, Metropolitan and a few Labour controlled and County Councils may have made equality improvement progress but there was little evidence of change among the many district councils. There is no evidence that there was any systematic attempt by FRS to engage in equality improvement.

The Commission for Racial Equality (CRE) had argued prophetically in 1979 that a drive towards racial equality without enthusiastic and publicly expressed support from the government was unlikely to be successful (Clarke and Speeden 2001), something which was not forthcoming after the general election of 1979. Attitudes changed somewhat during the Major administration of 1997 with a sustained campaign for and the passage of the DDA in 1995. In the absence of a favourable national political and policy environment, systematic equality improvement in the public sector was to say the least patchy.

Equality Management After Macpherson

The Macpherson report injected the idea of institutional discrimination into mainstream public policy discourse (MacPherson 1999). The Race Relations (Amendment) Act 2000, which followed Macpherson, marked an important innovation in the legal framework. It placed much of what had been up to then advisory and voluntary on to a statutory footing. The Act extended the positive provisions of the Race Relations Act 1976 to cover all the activities of all public authorities. It made important extensions to public authority duties and to the duties of the governing bodies of schools. Similar statutory duties were created for disability by the Disability Discrimination Act 2005 and for gender by the Equality Act 2006. These duties were divided into a general duty and specific duties. In particular, it was the specific duties that meshed with the new local government regulatory regime. Specific duties required policy development, impact assessment and the setting of equality improvement objectives (Neckles 2015).

From 1977 to 1995, the CRE had carried out more than 50 formal investigations into direct and indirect discrimination. A number of these had targeted local authority housing policy and practice and some aspects of the health service (Clarke and Speeden 2001: 25). There was a belief that the law, the requirements of a finding of discrimination and direct intervention by the CRE would change the behaviour both of the investigated organisation and organisations of a similar kind (Clarke and Speeden 2001). Fire brigades, as they were then, did not get a mention.

The formal investigation-based approach had very limited success, and it was recognised that there was a need for policy tools, which could change management practice in public service provision. In 1995, the CRE pioneered a 'total quality management' (TQM) approach to the improvement of equality policy and practice both for local authorities and private business.

In examining a range of models for policymaking and organisational change, the TQM approach provided an interesting model for cultural change in organisations that could provide a framework for equality management and improvement. The local government standard *Race Equality Means Quality* (Commission for Racial Equality 1995) was adopted by many authorities as an improvement tool. This approach became the basis for further work on an ESLG, which would deliver a unified approach for working on equality in Local Government.

In 1999, a consortium consisting of the Employers Organisation for Local Government, the three equality commissions and the Audit Commission working with the Centre for Local Policy Studies began to work on a unified standard for Local Government (DIALOG 2001, 2006). The work coincided with the publication of the Macpherson report, and the ESLG was launched in 2001 just after the passage of the Race Relations Amendment Act. The cooperation between the partners presaged the policy discussions that subsequently took place and which, resulted in the creation of the Equality and Human Rights Commission and then the 2010 Equality Act. The principal concern in developing the Standard was that a unified structure for implementing equalities should recognise the equal significance of each of the equality strands that it was trying to bring together.[1]

---

[1] The author was part of the team that developed the Equality Standard for Local Government.

Best Value assessments were introduced by the 1997 Labour Government. The Standard was launched in 2001 and became a Best Value Performance Indicator in April 2002 alongside indicators developed by the Commission for Racial Equality.[2] This meant that managers and staff within local government had to make major efforts to get to grips with the Standard and the work that it entailed. Implementing the Standard formed part of an ongoing agenda for change, which would take on board new elements (sexual orientation, age) over the next 5 years.

Subsequently, the Comprehensive Performance Assessments (CPA) attempted to encourage local authorities to adopt a more rigorous approach to performance management. CPA encouraged a self-assessment approach and brought the Equality Standard into the general framework for performance management and business planning. The clear intention was to bring equality into the 'mainstream' of policy development and management.

The ESLG was developed to take account of the changing context of local governance and the pressures for improvement imposed by central government. The Standard had both to fit with the modernising agenda for local government and also had to provide a systematic approach to managing equality that was capable of addressing patterns of institutional discrimination and provide demonstrable evidence of change.

Equality Improvement

The concept of equality improvement as a continuous process encompasses a range of changes in the way an organisation is managed and operates, leading first to output changes and (hopefully) then to outcome changes. Key principles which would lead to specific action included:

- Commitment to change at the level of the whole organisation
- Comprehensive approach to equality policy development and action planning
- Determination of service-relevant population groups/categories
- Engagement/consultation with different sections of the population
- Equality impact/risk assessment
- Commitment to self-assessment
- Commitment to equal service delivery for different population categories
- Performance management
- Equality in employment for different population categories
- Management structure and accountability in relation to all of the above

(DIALOG 2001)

---

[2] These were Best Value Performance Indicators 2a and 2b.

FRS Engagement with Equality Improvement

FRSs were pulled into the general local government modernisation and improvement process by the Bains et al. (2002) report, the 2004 Fire Services Act and the regulation regimes supervised by the Audit Commission. A 1999 thematic review of equality in FRS refers to a speech made by the then Home Secretary, Jack Straw, in which:

He described the fire services record to date in the field of equality as *unacceptable.*

> The Government wanted a fire service that looked like Britain in all of its diversity. That could only strengthen the service and its reputation. It was time for the service to stop making excuses and to set its house in order. (Home Office 1999, p.11)

A top-down approach was adopted by Government. The Home Office produced an equality action planning document (Home Office 2000) with an emphasis on Chief Fire Officer leadership and both on equality in employment and community engagement. This was followed at the end of 2001 by a second action plan, this time sponsored by the Department of Transport, Local Government and the Regions (DTLR). Both plans were produced in conjunction with the existing equality commissions and a number of equality campaign groups. In 2006, the new Department of Communities and Local Government (DCLG) produced a case study document indicating what action had been taken in English FRS. The case studies covered the following policy areas:

- Tackling bullying and harassment
- Respecting religious customs and beliefs
- Respecting sexual orientation
- Recruiting women firefighters
- Recruiting people with disabilities
- Recruiting black and minority ethnic (BME) firefighters
- Retaining and supporting people with disabilities
- Promoting community cohesion
- Engaging with hard to reach groups
- Partnership working for equality and diversity
- Mainstreaming equality and diversity
- Increasing understanding of faith issues in the Fire and Rescue Service
- A national initiative

(DCLG 2006).

Although there was a distinct focus on equality in employment, there were several examples of an emergent approach to community safety work with a range of communities. The examples were drawn from less than 10 of the 47 existing FRS.

The document also contains key forward looking recommendations:

- Adapting the Local Government Equality Standard for Fire and Rescue Services and benchmarking the results

- Review of the recruitment, progression and retention targets for BME (black and minority ethnic) groups and women
- Including diversity in the Comprehensive Performance Assessment framework for FRS

(DCLG 2006).

Disappointment with progress, however, was expressed by both the Select Committee (House of Commons, 2006) and the Commission for Racial Equality (2006) about a lack of *consistent* progress. The parliamentary committee was principally concerned with employment targets:

> FRS were set a target to achieve 9 per cent of uniformed operational staff being women and 3.6 per cent of uniformed and non-uniformed combined being ethnic minorities by 31 March 2004. None of these targets were met, as only 2.4 per cent of the workforce were women and 2.6 per cent were from ethnic minorities by the 2004 deadline. (House of Commons 2006, p.44)

FRS argued that the targets were impossible to achieve in the existing recruitment conditions (House of Commons 2006). No connection was made by the parliamentarians between the post-2004 emphasis on fire protection and community safety and equality policy and practice.

Change in FRS Approaches to Equality Improvement 2004–2010

A combination of factors encouraged FRS to develop both a broader and more systematic approach to equality policy and practice. The three sets of drivers broadly defined in the introduction to the chapter attained a more precise form at this time, which can be characterised as follows:

- A series of new statutes with positive duty elements and the requirement to produce equality schemes and action plans overseen by the three equality commissions
- A new FRS statutory framework in the 2004 Act that emphasised systematic risk assessment in relation to prevention and community safety leading to an examination of the variety of risks faced by different population categories and social groups
- A regulatory regime inspected by the Audit Commission (in the CPA and then the Comprehensive Area Assessment (CAA)) that contained an important equality element leading to the adoption of improved performance management techniques across all aspects of employment practice and service delivery
- The development of the ESLG, which provided a clear and coherent, level-based framework for working on equality improvement

Following the passage of the Race Relations (Amendment) Act of 2000, all public service bodies were required to produce a race equality scheme. Subsequently they were required to produce both gender and disability equality schemes. From 2004, the principal policy and planning document that each Fire Authority had a statutory duty to produce was the Integrated Risk Management Plan (IRMP).

In parallel with the production of equality schemes and action plans, local authorities and FRS were required to demonstrate to the Audit Commission that they were integrating equality improvement work into the general management planning of their organisation.

The equality improvement task faced by all FRS was to produce assessments of risk that lined up with the duties previously described. One of the means by which many FRS chose to structure this work was to adopt and work to the ESLG as was recommended by the DCLG (DCLG 2006). Both the contents of the race equality scheme and the level of the ESLG achieved became Best Value indicators in 2002. Public service bodies were required to report against these indicators providing another incentive for FRS to adopt the Standard. Using the Standard complemented the statutory requirement to produce Race and then disability and gender equality schemes. Work with the Standard also supported positive community safety assessments during CPA and CAA inspections, which facilitated FRS engagement (see for example Audit Commission 2005).

The exact number of English FRSs that did detailed work using ESLG is difficult to determine. Although all FRSs were supposed to submit a self-assessed evaluation against Best Value indicators 2a and 2b, there was no systematic national-level test of the value of these self-assessments. Twelve out of the then 47 services requested Equality Mark assessments, which were organised by the author and carried out by a team of equality consultants who had undertaken training specific to the work. The proportion of FRSs presenting themselves for external assessment was at the end of 2008 much higher than for local authorities.

The ESLG required that organisations work through five levels of activity. These levels would take them from systematic corporate policy making and commitment to equality improvement, through impact assessment and action planning to actual change in organisational behaviour and measurable outcomes in terms of service delivery and employment practice.

All 12 FRSs that sought external evaluation asked to be assessed at Level 3 of ESLG. This required that the organisation had been through Levels 1 and 2, which were the commitment and policy development and action planning stages. Level 2 had required that the organisation had:

- Engaged in an impact and needs/requirements assessment
- Engaged in consultation with designated community, staff and stakeholders
- Engaged in the development of information and monitoring systems
- Engaged in an equality action planning process for employment, pay and service delivery
- Engaged in developing a system of self-assessment, scrutiny and audit

(DIALOG 2001/2006).

For an assessment at Level 3, a FRS had to show that:

- It has completed a full and systematic consultation process with designated community, staff and stakeholder groups.
- It has set equality objectives for employment, pay and service delivery based on impact and needs/requirements assessment and consultation.
- Equality objectives have been translated into action plans with specific targets.
- It is developing information and monitoring systems that allow it to assess progress in achieving targets.
- Action on achieving targets has started.

(DIALOG 2001/2006).

All 12 FRSs produced detailed self-assessment documents indicating that the required criteria had been met. Assessors tested the self-assessments in 2 days of interviews with a sample of FRS staff that included senior managers, equality improvement staff and front-line firefighters.

All assessed FRSs could provide good evidence of Level 1 attainment. The key area in which FRSs had diverged from what was intended in the ESLG was their approach to equality impact assessment and action planning. At first view, it seemed that FRSs had not understood the purpose of equality impact assessment. This was to assess where population categories designated by equality legislation (broadly people from minorities, women and disabled people) were not receiving equal treatment in terms of service delivery and employment opportunities. On the whole, formally designated equality impact assessment reports provided by FRSs did not provide evidence of detailed examination of the equality impact of FRSs practice. Closer examination of the way in which FRSs had used the Standard revealed that substantive equality impact assessment, in the way intended by the Standard, was being done in the development of IRMPs.

> Equality Mark assessment showed a key difference between local authorities and FRS. Local authorities used equality impact assessments in a number of ways. Principally they were used to review the impact of service delivery procedures on different equality categories/strands; asking, for example, whether a particular service was reaching a particular category of people or whether a service was meeting the needs of that category. Many local authorities assembled detailed bodies of evidence to support the findings of their assessments. Fire services have not, on the whole, used equality impact assessments in this way. They have tended to use them to "future proof" new policies; that is, to see whether a new policy is likely to have an adverse equality impact when introduced. (Clarke and Kaleem 2010, p.14)

FRSs were, therefore, engaged in a type of equality impact assessment via their assessments of the safety risks to various population categories, the vulnerability of these categories to harm from fire and, for example, from road traffic collisions.

That FRSs did the work in this manner is not surprising. During the same period that FRSs were grappling with a new regulatory regime that included a multilayered approach to equality improvement, the DCLG funded a major programme of home fire risk safety checks during which nearly 2 million homes were visited and 2.5 million smoke alarms installed between 2000 and 2008 (DCLG 2009a). A parallel Fire Prevention Grant (FPG) provided other wider opportunities.

> The FPG enabled FRSs to try out new *innovative* and *creative* initiatives and activities that
> they previously would not have been able to do. (DCLG 2009a, p.5)

These initiatives included both work done by FRS alone and by FRS in a widened
range of partnerships with both the voluntary sector and other public sector service
organisations, particularly local authorities. FRS work included fire safety checks
with people who have sensory loss, minority groups and individuals at risk of
domestic violence. In particular, it allowed the employment of specialist advocates
and work with young people in areas other than fire risk such as driving safety
(DCLG 2009a). Arguably, the FPG also encouraged the development of the simple
fire risk check into the more ambitious home safety assessment. Other partnership
bids for grant funding based on this broader notion of risk assessment thus became
plausible (Clarke 2016).

One FRS from the north-east of England had identified a range of at risk categories of people, which only partially coincided with the categories identified in the
then current (2007) equality legislation.[3] The FRS found that:

- Single males were disproportionately affected by chip pan fires. A programme of
  free replacement of chip pans with deep fat fryers contributed to almost halving
  their incidence between 2003 and 2006.
- Teenagers, both male and female, were disproportionately vulnerable to injury
  and death in road traffic accidents. The FRS has an extensive youth work programme that attempts to reduce teenage death and injury through re-education.
- BME groups and asylum seekers were disproportionately vulnerable to death
  and injury by fire. This has been specifically recognised by the FRS both as an
  equality and cohesion issue and a number of initiatives were undertaken to
  reduce such deaths and injuries.
- Older and disabled people were vulnerable to different kinds of accidents in their
  homes both from fires and from slips and falls. The preventative action that was
  taken not only reduced injury and distress to older and disabled people; it probably supported savings in health care expenditure.
- An advocate programme that recruited officers with specific skills and attributes
  worked towards better service delivery for specific groups including BME people and disabled and older people. Work was also done on alcohol and drug
  dependence.
- A community cohesion strategy was developed from revised risk assessments for
  BME community groups.
- Employment and training targets were set. (CLPS 2007)

The 12 FRSs that were assessed in 2007 and 2008 met the Level 3 service delivery criteria at the in terms of *outputs*. They had undertaken thorough self-assessment,
detailed policy development, had engaged with equality impact assessment and set
out action plans for service delivery, employment and procurement. The Equality

---

[3] This FRS was ahead of the equality curve because the 'at risk' categories that were identified
would have been covered by the range of protected characteristics defined by the 2010 Equality
Act.

Mark reports all contained agreed sets of improvements that FRS needed to undertake and also outlined what was required to reach the next Level 4 of the Standard. Moving to Level 4 and then Level 5 would have required the FRSs to go beyond the action planning and target setting stage and be able to demonstrate actual equality improvement *outcomes*.

At a national level the fire service set out a long-term commitment in a ten-year equality strategy in 2008:

> Equality and Diversity are key issues for the Fire and Rescue Service. They must drive how we treat each other as members of the Service; how we treat each of our customers; how we interact with the diverse communities we serve, and how we deliver our services to those communities. To be an effective Service our policies, practices and procedures must be fair, providing equality of opportunity to all employees and an appropriate and effective service to all parts of the community. (DCLG 2008, p.9)

In parallel with this national declaration, a decision was taken to develop a FRS-specific equality management tool, and between 2009 and 2012, a *Fire and Rescue Equality Framework* was refined and published (Local Government Association 2012). In effect, this was a simplified version of the new *Equality Framework for Local Government* (Improvement and Development Agency 2009) which was in turn based on the ESLG. Both were level-based standards but had three levels rather than five: 'developing', 'achieving' and 'excellent'. Both frameworks developed a peer assessment model where the level reached was assessed by a team drawn, in the FRS case, from staff and councillors from other FRSs and Fire and Rescue Authorities (FRAs).

Austerity and 'Light Touch' Regulation

One of the last legislative achievements of the 2005 Labour Government was the Equality Act 2010. It replaced previous legislation that had provided for race, gender and disability discrimination and enlarged the list of what were called 'protected characteristics'. Age, gender reassignment, marriage and civil partnership, pregnancy and maternity, religion or belief and sexual orientation were added to the three existing categories. The Act retained the same internal structure as previous legislation. There was a general duty not to discriminate either directly or indirectly. At the time of the 2010 General election, the detail of a specific Public Sector Equality Duty (PSED) was still to be decided. The Coalition Government was not enthusiastic about the detail of public sector regulation, and although there was no chance that they would repeal the 2010, they began to remove much of the supporting framework (Neckles 2015). The Audit Commission, for example, was wound down in favour of a much vaunted 'light touch' approach to public service regulation.

Initiatives such as the Red Tape Challenge removed much of the protective detail from the working of the Equality Act (Neckles 2015). The PSED emerged from these processes shorn also of some important provision. The only substantive specific duties that attached to the PSED were a requirement to publish: *'specific and measurable' equality objectives but only every four years. [and] that the information published must be 'in a manner accessible to the public'* (Neckles 2015). No requirement for self-assessment, equality impact assessment or equality schemes remained. Austerity and budget reductions meant also that many FRSs lost dedicated equality staff.

Despite these changes equality improvement has remained part of the way in which FRSs see themselves. Twelve FRSs have been judged to be either achieving or excellent in relation to the *Fire and Rescue Service Equality Framework* (LGA 2016). Four of these completed Level 3 of the ESLG which means that twenty FRSs have self-assessed and put themselves forward for external assessment since 2008.

Engagement with the Equality Framework for FRS

To qualitatively test both progress in equality improvement and conformity with the (admittedly limited) specific duties, five FRSs that had achieved 'excellent' against the FRS Equality Framework were qualitatively compared against five FRSs that showed no indication of having engaged with it. The FRS were taken from family groups 2 and 4 (DCLG 2009b).[4] Comparison was based on the range of written documentation accessible to the public. The documents that were sought included a basic equality statement, a more developed equality policy, equality impact policy or guidance, actual impact assessment reports, equality consultation reports, a communities' strategy, a detailed communications strategy, work force profiling, an equality contact point, dedicated equality staff and a recent (post-2012) equality self-assessment.

It was evident that there was a difference between the two categories.[5] The FRS that had achieved an excellent rating in the peer assessment process had made available a wider range of documentation explaining the nature of their equality improvement strategy and what actions they were taking to implement the strategy. They were providing a consistent range of information across most of the categories indicated above. Equally clear was that the FRS not engaged with the peer assessment had continued to develop their equality improvement work. There were publications and evidence of work from all the FRSs. The second group, however, did not show the same kind of consistency and breadth of information provision as the first.

FRSs peer assessed as 'excellent' also seemed to have better developed communications strategies, making more and wider ranging documentation available to service users. A wide range of published equality documentation is important

---

[4]For comparative purposes, DCLG divided FRS into five family groups on the basis of variation in population concentrations and geographical diversity.

[5]It must be emphasised that this is a judgement based on a limited qualitative assessment. Further more detailed research is required to find out if quality of service matches quality of documentation.

because it provides a set of criteria against which FRSs can be assessed and held accountable. If an FRS claims to have carried out recent equality impact assessments or a recent equality self-assessment councillors, other public sector and voluntary sector organisations can see what the FRS is claiming to have done and can confirm or challenge the claims. Where documentation is non-existent or sparse, there is at least an indication that not much has been going on by way of equality improvement work and it is more difficult to set up a change dialogue. The absence of documentation should indicate to responsible local politicians that they need to interrogate their service about what kind of equality efforts are being made.

A principal demonstrable example of equality improvement has been the development of fire safety checks into more broad-based home safety assessments. The recruitment of specialist advocates with specific remits related to some of 2010 Equality Act protected groups has been a feature of many fire and rescue services. Eight out of the ten FRSs examined had either paid or voluntary community advocates working on fire and general home safety; all five of the FRSs assessed as 'excellent' operated such a system together with three from the other group.

One north-west FRS made a bid for a Migrant Impact Fund grant in 2009 to deliver both fire safety work and public service information to eastern European migrants. A successful partnership was set up with their local authorities and domestic violence third-sector organisations employing bilingual advocates. It provided home safety assessments for migrant households and also signposted access to local public services (Clarke 2016). The same FRS has recently entered into partnership with the NHS and another north-west FRS to provide health information and risk assessments for older people.[6]

In relation to improving equality in employment, the situation is complex. Recruitment patterns have meant that it was impossible to meet some of the more ambitious targets for overall equality in employment. But where figures have been published, the detail does show some limited achievement. The London Fire Brigade has kept detailed employment records since 2002. Between that year and 2015, there was a proportional increase in BME operational firefighters from 6.79 to 12.18%. For operational women firefighters during the same period the proportion has increased from 2.13 to 6.24%. The proportions for non-operational employees over the same period were from 22.65 to 26.3% for BME staff and for women a decline from 49.95 to 44.24%. There was an increase for both groups in terms of successful applications over 2011 and 2013. Promotions for both BME and women staff recorded improved percentages between 2011 and 2014 (as against applications). Just over 3% of operational staff (142) were recorded as disabled in 2013/2014 with a slightly higher percentage identifying as LGB (188) (LFEPA 2015).

Figures for London show an increase over the first decade of this century except in overall female staffing. The proportion of BME operational firefighters, which was a main policy focus of the two Ken Livingstone London administrations, has increased. Recent recruitment figures do show targets set in 2004/2005 finally being met.[7]

---

[6] Personal communication with responsible FRS officers and access to unpublished documents
[7] This information was obtained when the author and colleagues were conducting an equality

Comparing 2012/13 to 2013/14, the proportion of BME joiners increased from 18.6 per cent (11 out of 59) to 28.9 per cent (11 out of 38), and the proportion of women joiners increased from 39.0 percent (23 out of 59) to 39.5 per cent (15 out of 38) (LFEPA 2015, p13).

Other FRSs have made figures available over a narrower and more recent date ranges and indicate that while some progress has been made, both recruitment and appointment figures do not indicate a real shift towards proportional employment in operational roles relative to local population distributions. Women's employment in support roles often shows female majorities (see for example Greater Manchester FRS 2016) but limited progress has been made in operational recruitment. A number of FRSs have developed positive action policies and pursued recruitment initiatives and provided advice and support on physical fitness (see for example Tyne and Wear FRS 2016). Despite this recruitment to operational roles has, on the whole, remained below targets set in 2009 (Waters 2009). Further research is required to determine the reasons.

Conclusion

At the turn of the century, FRSs were viewed as white male organisations that were exclusionary, exhibiting racist, sexist and homophobic behaviours. This chapter has taken a historical developmental route to examining the way in which fire and rescue services have improved fair and equal treatment of service users and worked on positive equality approaches to staff recruitment, retention and promotion.

Equality policy improvement in relation to service delivery involves impact assessment in relation to population categories covered by equality law. It also requires risk assessment to determine whether those population categories that might be more vulnerable to fire injury and death than other categories belong to the categories protected by equality legislation. Equality in staff recruitment, development and promotion presents a parallel set of problems; it requires sufficient levels of recruitment to allow employment from underrepresented population categories and attraction of enough (qualified) individuals from those categories as well as genuinely open recruitment processes.

This chapter started with a commentary on the concepts of equality and diversity, equal opportunities and equality of outcome. It then briefly explored the emergence of equality policy and management between 1965 and the Macpherson report of 1999.

The section that followed focused on the period of major legislative, regulatory and policy development between 2000 and 2010. The introduction of the ESLG and its use by FRS was discussed and detailed. During engagement with ESLG, FRSs

assessment for the GLA in 2004. The aim for both BME groups and women was to approach London population proportions. The original policy documents are no longer available to the author.

produced a range of outputs, particularly a wide range of policy documents relating to both service delivery and employment and to the setting of equality targets in both areas. Twelve out of 47 FRSs sought external assessment of their ESLG achievements. It was argued that change was driven by:

- A series of new statutes with positive duty elements and the requirement to produce equality schemes and action plans overseen by the three equality commissions
- A new FRS statutory framework in the 2004 Act that emphasised systematic risk assessment in relation to prevention and community safety leading to an examination of the variety of risks faced by different population categories and social groups
- A regulatory regime inspected by the Audit Commission (in the CPA and then the CAA) that contained an important equality element leading to the adoption of improved performance management techniques across all aspects of employment practice and service delivery
- The development of the ESLG which provided a clear and coherent level-based framework for working on equality improvement

The last section of this chapter then examined what has happened during the more recent periods of Coalition and Conservative government after 2010 when ESLG was replaced by a dedicated fire service equality framework that was subject to peer review and assessment rather than external validation. The detailed regulatory regimes of the previous decade were replaced by 'light touch' oversight. The targets set for positive equality action in service delivery have been followed through by many FRSs both in the way that risk assessment has taken on some features of equality impact assessment and in the way FRSs have taken up or created equality-oriented initiatives and partnership projects. The extent to which this kind of development extends across all FRSs is not clear and requires further research. Equality improvement in employment outcomes appears to have been much more limited. Women support staff are in a majority in some FRSs and there is evidence to suggest that FRS have continued with positive attempts to recruit operational firefighters from underrepresented categories. There has, however, been limited success for reasons that are complex and are not reducible to either direct or indirect discrimination, clearly this also requires further research.

References

Arneson, R. (2015). *Equality of opportunity, the Stanford encyclopedia of philosophy* (summer 2015 edition), Stanford: Stanford.

Audit Commission. (2005). *Fire and rescue comprehensive performance assessment: Merseyside fire and rescue authority*. London: Audit Commission.

Bagilhole, B. (1993). Managing to be fair: Implementing equal opportunities in a local authority. *Local Government Studies, 19*(2), 163–175.

Bagilhole, B. (1997). *Equal opportunities and social policy*. London: Longman.

Bain G., Lyons M., & Young M. (2002). The future of the fire service; reducing risks saving lives: The independent review of the Fire Service London TSO.

Clarke, J. (2016). Beyond authority: Public value, innovation and entrepreneurship in a UK fire and rescue service. In J. Liddle (Ed.), *New perspectives on research, policy & practice in public entrepreneurship* (pp. 213–236). Bradford: Emerald.

Clarke, J., & Kaleem, N. (2010). Equality, vulnerability, risk and service delivery: Equality improvement in fire and rescue services. *International Fire Service Journal of Leadership and Management, 4*(2), 13–22.

Clarke, J., & Speeden, S. (2001). Then and now: Change for the better? A review of 25 years work by the Commission for Racial Equality, London: Commission for Racial Equality Cleveland Fire Brigade Equality Mark Level 3 Assessment and Validation Report, unpublished.

Collier, R. (1998). *Equality in managing service delivery*. Buckingham: Open University Press.

Commission for Racial Equality. (1995). *Racial equality means quality*. London: Commission for Racial Equality.

Commission for Racial Equality. (2006). *Memorandum by the Commission for Racial Equality*. London: HMG.

Daniel, W. W. (1968). *Racial discrimination in England: Based on the PEP report*. London: Penguin.

DCLG. (2006). *Equality and diversity matters, examples of good practice to promote equality and diversity in the fire and rescue service*. London: DCLG.

DCLG. (2008). *Fire and rescue service equality and diversity strategy 2008 to 2018*. Wetherby: Communities and Local Government Publications.

DCLG. (2009a). *Final evaluation of the home fire risk check grant and fire prevention grant programmes*. London: DCLG.

DCLG. (2009b). *Review of fire and rescue service response times, fire research series 1*. London: DCLG.

DIALOG. (2001). *Equality standard for local government*. London: DIALOG.

DIALOG. (2006). *Equality standard for local government (revised)*. London: DIALOG.

DTLR. (2001). *Toward diversity II commitment to cultural change: The second fire service equal opportunities action plan*. London: Department of Transport Local Government and the Regions.

Fire Brigades Union. (2006). Firefighter magazine, Kingston-upon-Thames.

Greater Manchester FRS. (2016). http://www.manchesterfire.gov.uk/about_us /equality_and_ diversity/gmfrs-workforce-profile/.

Hepple, B. A., Coussey, M., & Choudhury, T. (2000). *Equality, a new framework: Report of the independent review of the enforcement of UK anti-discrimination legislation*. Oxford: Hart.

Home Office. (1999). *Equality and fairness in the fire service*. London: Home Office.

Home Office. (2000). *Towards diversity promoting cultural change: Fire service equality action plan*. London: Home Office.

House of Commons. (2006). *Communities and local government committee fire and rescue service fourth report of session 2005–06*. London: HMG.

Improvement and Development Agency. (2009). *Equality framework for local government*. London: IDeA.

Kandola, R., Fullerton, J., & Ahmed, Y. (1995). Managing diversity: Succeeding where equal opportunities have failed. *Equal Opportunities Review, 50*, 31–36.

LFEPA. (2015). *Employment monitoring data and publication of results for 2013/14*. London: LFEPA.

Local Government Association. (2012). *Fire and rescue service equality framework and peer challenge toolkit*. London: LGA.

Local Government Association. (2016). http://www.local.gov.uk/peer-challenges/-/journal_ content/56/10180/3510141/ARTICLE.

Macpherson, W. (1999). *The Stephen Lawrence inquiry, cm. 4262-I*. London: TSO.

Mid and West Wales Wales FRS Annual Equality Report 1st April 2012 to 31 March 2013, Mid and West Wales FRS: Knighton.

Miles, R. (1982). *Racism and migrant labour*. London: Routledge, Chapman & Hall.

Neckles, L. (2015). The effectiveness of the race and disability public sector equality duties as positive legal duties and legal accountability tools, PhD, Edgehill University.

Ross, R., & Schneider, R. (1992). *From equality to diversity: Business case for equal opportunity*. London: Pitman.

Stonewall. (2016). *Top 100 employers: The Stonewall equality index*. London: Stonewall.

Thornton, P., & Lunt, N. (1993). Employment for disabled people social obligation or individual responsibility? Social policy reports, no 2, Social Policy Research Unit, York: University of York.

Tyne and Wear FRS. (2016). http://www.twfire.gov.uk/recruitment/firefighters/positive-action-events/#.WAnH9OArLIU.

UK Fire Resources Group. (2014). http://www.fireservice.co.uk/recruitment/physical.

Waters, A. (2009). Positive action in firefighter recruitment, Networking Women in the Fire Service.

Dr. Julian Clarke has a social sciences background including a PhD in social anthropology. Teaching and research originally focused on ethnicity, race, migration and equality policy. This eventually led to work with the Commission for Racial Equality and the Local Government Association. He was a member of a team that developed the Equality Standard for Local Government and a subsequent assessment programme. A number of FRS took up the Equality Standard and were assessed against the framework. A research interest in FRS management grew out of this work focused primarily on public service partnership and the creation of public value.

Chapter 12
Governance Matters

Catherine Farrell

Introduction

This chapter focuses on the governance of the Fire and Rescue Service (FRS). This topic is an under-researched area. The Fire and Rescue Authority (FRA) is effectively the governing body or board for the Fire and Rescue Service (FRS) and their role in governance is an under-researched area. Very little is known about how governance operates in practice within Fire and Rescue Authorities. This chapter examines the governance of the Fire and Rescue Service and brings this topic area under greater scrutiny.

The vast majority of academic work on the fire and rescue focuses on the modernisation of the service after the Bain Report of 2002 (e.g. Andrews 2010; Matheson et al. 2011) and there is some literature on changes within the service including the extent of preventative work which the service has engaged in over time (e.g. Childs et al. 2004). Murphy and Greenhalgh's (2013) research is on performance management within the service and how performance can be improved. However, within the existing academic literature, governance is an under-researched issue and it is not clear how effective Fire and Rescue Authorities are in leading the service. No research has been conducted on how the service is governed or the operation of the existing stakeholder model of governance which operates in the Fire and Rescue Service. This chapter aims to review governance, bring together evidence on its operation mainly from professional sources and present some of the issues around the existing governance arrangements and alternatives to this.

C. Farrell (✉)
Professor of Public Management, Department of Social Sciences,
University of South Wales, Pontypridd, UK
e-mail: catherine.farrell@southwales.ac.uk

© Springer International Publishing AG 2018
P. Murphy, K. Greenhalgh (eds.), *Fire and Rescue Services*,
DOI 10.1007/978-3-319-62155-5_12

Good Governance

The board model for leading public, private and third sector institutions is widely prevalent across the UK. This model separates the leadership of institutions from those responsible for their day-to-day operation. The board, which typically comprises individuals from various backgrounds and with a range of different kinds of expertise, is primarily responsible for the overall conduct and governance of the institution and its strategic position in the medium and long term. The person with responsibility for the proper functioning of the institution on a day-to-day basis, who is typically referred to as the Chief Executive Officer (CEO), or Chief Officer, is normally a member of the board. Given the significance of the board's responsibility for leadership, the constitution of public sector boards and the background and expertise of board members have received comparatively little attention by researchers.

The governing board features in many organisations and services. In the Fire and Rescue Service, the board is called the Fire and Rescue Authority; in education, the board is the school governing body; and in health, the board is the health board. Third sector and voluntary organisations also have boards and these may be called 'trustee boards' or non-profit boards with members referred to as 'trustees'. Private companies also have boards and in this sector, they are called boards of directors. Cornforth's research focuses on boards across public and non-profit organisations and specifically, the role of the board (Cornforth 2003). The chapter includes empirical studies on the operation of boards in practice. Farrell (2005) has reviewed the operation of school-governing bodies and the extent to which they are involved in strategic activities including leadership and decision-making. Key findings indicate that executives including head-teachers and others within the staff of a school are at least as involved as governing bodies. This finding is not unique – McNulty and Pettigrew's (1999) study of the operation of boards of directors in the private sector also indicates that board members could be more involved in strategic and leadership activities. More recently, Brown's (2014) paper on board member participation in practice reminds us of the importance of the need for individuals to agree in terms of the values of the organisation, the existence of trust and also positive group dynamics amongst other factors.

Many of the elements picked up by Brown (2014) are presented below. Good governance is dependent on the existence and effective operation of the following six principles:

Good governance is dependent on the existence and effective operation of:

1. The organisation's purpose and on outcomes for citizens and users
2. Performing effectively in clearly defined functions and roles
3. Promoting values for the whole organisation and demonstrating the values of good governance through behaviour
4. Taking informed, transparent decisions and managing risk
5. Developing the capacity and capability of the governing body to be effective
6. Engaging stakeholders and making accountability real

Ref – OPM and CIPFA, 2004, *The Good Governance Standard for Public Services*.

These elements will be used in the review of governance in the Fire and Rescue Service presented in this chapter.

The Stakeholder Model of Governance

The Fire and Rescue Service has its roots within both local governments. Before the Second World War, the fire service was organised and delivered by local government and in some areas, the responsibility was delegated to the police service. During the war, the fire service was nationalised and it was decided that at the end of the war, the service would be returned to local authorities. In 1947, the Fire Services Act became law and local councils had a fire department to administer. At this point in time, the main service delivered was extinguishing fires, and very little was included about the other functions of the fire service. An element of prevention was included in their responsibilities in which on request, the fire service could provide fire prevention advice. Over time, as evidenced in other chapters of this text, the preventative aspect of the work of the Fire and Rescue Services has grown and it was formally included in the Fire and Rescue Services Act 2004.

Today, FRAs are responsible for leading the service including fire emergencies, promoting fire safety, dealing with road traffic accidents and other emergency situations such as flooding, although this is not a statutory field of responsibility. In England, there are 46 Fire and Rescue Services and three in Wales. The parent department in England up until very recently (2016) was the Department for Communities and Local Government and responsibility has now transferred to the Home Office. In Wales, where the service has been devolved since 2006, responsibility lies with the Welsh Government.

Under the Fire and Rescue Services Act 2004, the Fire and Rescue Authority for an area in England is a non-metropolitan county council is the Fire and Rescue Authority for the county or a non-metropolitan district council for an area for which there is no county council, the London Fire and Emergency Planning Authority or the Council of the Isles of Scilly. In Wales, the FRA is either a county or county borough council or a merged group of these councils. Under the 2004 legislation, FRAs have four key responsibilities:

- Extinguishing fires in their area
- Protecting life and property in the event of fires in their area
- Rescuing and protecting people in the event of a road traffic collision
- Rescuing and protecting people in the event of other emergencies

Under the National Frameworks, FRAs have to be accountable for the service which they provide.

In line with the history of the service, the current model of governance features a membership drawn from local government. It is councillors elected to the local authorities which make up the Fire and Rescue Service (FRS) who are then 'appointed' to the Fire and Rescue Authority (FRA). In England, most local authorities have their own Fire and Rescue Authority and where this is not the case, the Authority is drawn from a number of local council areas. The members of the FRA are drawn from their 'parent' councils on the basis of their size and in the majority of cases, political representation. Thus, in the FRS in South Wales, there are 24 members drawn proportionately from ten local authorities on the basis of size, their political representation and other factors which are deemed relevant. This may include gender, for example, and local authorities will use a range of different factors to identify those members from their areas who will sit on the FRA.

This is a stakeholder model of governance where those with a 'stake' or 'interest' in the service are part of the governing board. Citizens elect their local councillors and it is a group of these members who have a seat around the governance table. This approach was broadly the one which operated in the police service until its replacement with the elected approach in 2012. Those in governance roles in the Fire and Rescue Service are a group of those who have been elected to local government and their interest or stake is built on their foundation as local members. The stakeholder approach in this context is based on a democratic model involving local councillors who have been elected by citizens to be directly involved in decision-making and governance.

A key issue relevant to the governance of the FRAs is the funding of the service. Under the existing model of governance, FRAs are funded from their parent authorities which each levy an additional amount of money for the Fire and Rescue Service. This source of funding, together with the governing board made up of local councillors, means that FRAs operate independently from direct central government control. They therefore cannot be managed and controlled by central government and there is a democratic element to their constituency as their members are directly elected local councillors. Board members therefore cannot be appointed by central government unlike the majority of public boards and health boards. This is an important background to the existing governance model which operates in the FRAs in England and Wales and until recently, in Scotland. It means that control lies within the board and the board is therefore solely responsible as the decision-making body for the FRS.

Governance Under the Spotlight

The governance of the Fire and Rescue Service has not received a great deal of attention within the academic literature. One of the first reviews into the operation of the Fire and Rescue Service was led by Sir George Bain in 2002 (Bain 2002) and the findings of this fed into the Fire and Rescue Services Act 2004. This Act, which repealed the Fire Services Act of 1947, was intended to deliver a modernised service responsive to the demands of the twenty-first century. It introduced new measures to force Fire and Rescue Authorities to act in accordance with the Fire and Rescue

National Framework ('the Framework') when carrying out their duties. This Framework was put in place by the Secretary of State and it set out the central government's priorities and objectives for the Fire and Rescue Services of England and Wales.

The modernisation of the Fire and Rescue Service has been on the agenda of a number of governments for some time and part of this has been focused on reforming the model of governance. This agenda has been particularly evident in England. A series of reports published under the banner 'Fire Futures' reflect similar discourses to those that have driven reform within education in England and also the police service in England and Wales. The reports include an examination of delivery models (Milsted 2010), decentralisation and citizen empowerment (Robinson 2010), localism and accountability (De Savage 2010), efficiency, effectiveness and productivity review (Hood 2010) and an options review for the service. Focusing particularly on governance, DeSavage (2010, p.5) proposes an alternative model of governance 'to develop nationally/adopt locally an alternative structure with a smaller number of authority members overall together with the inclusion of independents, to give a clearer voice to local priorities in line with other public service models'. It suggests that FRAs could identify mechanisms to enhance 'local community and independent involvement in scrutiny and governance structures'. One of the suggestions includes 'better representation for all tiers of local government and the private, third sector and even service management of the representative bodies' with the aim of enhancing local accountability as well as adding specific expertise to the governance arrangements.

In the 2012 National Framework for England, the need for FRAs to be accountable to their communities was highlighted. The key elements of this were the need for the FRA to hold the Chief Fire Officer to account for the delivery of the service, and also there needs to be 'arrangements in place to ensure that their decisions are open to scrutiny' (DCLG 2012, p15). In meeting this latter objective, FRAs must ensure transparency in data on aspects including performance and also the need to allow data comparisons between Fire and Rescue Services and other public services.

More recently, the governance of the Fire and Rescue Service came under the spotlight again in 2013 with the Knight review (Knight 2013). In this, the issues of governance and scrutiny were once again focused on and questions were asked about how effective the existing approach to governance was. The review concluded that the extent to which the FRA is effective in governance is patchy. It highlighted that FRAs have not 'fully embraced the 2012 National Framework requirements on governance and scrutiny and consequently the variety of structures that have been put in place do not seem to be effective'. In this report, scrutiny in some authorities is described as 'robust and independent' and in others too 'high level' to be meaningful. The report argues that:

> elected Police and Crime Commissioners were introduced because former Police Authorities
> ... were not seen as providing enough scrutiny and accountability to the public. A similar
> model for fire could clarify accountability arrangements and ensure more direct visibility to
> the electorate.

In terms of the key aspects of scrutiny and governance which are mentioned in the Knight (2013) review, the formal situation is one in which the Fire and Rescue Authority should hold their Chief Fire Officer/Chief Executive to account for the delivery of the Fire and Rescue Service was raised. Knight (2013) also recommended that FRAs should have arrangements in place to ensure decisions are open to scrutiny by citizens and others too. It is suggested too that the public needs to be able to access information in a way that enables them to compare the performance of their Fire and Rescue Service with others. The report was critical of the 46 FRAs 'different governance structures, senior leaders and organisational operational quirks does not make for a sensible delivery model' (Knight 2013) and put forward the need for greater 'interoperability' between emergency services including the Fire and Rescue Service, the police and the ambulance service. The report states that 'merging fire and rescue services with one or more of the other blue light services and/or sharing governance structures' could result in efficiencies overall. It is not clear how these governance arrangements would operate in practice or whether a single approach would be recommended for FRAs across England.

In England, there has once again been a recent focus on FRA governance. Launched in 2015, a consultation on the governance of the Fire and Rescue Service has outlined a range of different proposals for reforming governance including an extension of the police commissioner model, the enhancement of greater joint working between the police, fire and rescue and also the ambulance service under the authority of an emergency services commissioner (HM Government 2015). It seems from this consultation document that the there is a preference for an elected model of governance whereby 'the sharp focus of directly accountable leadership can play a critical role in securing better commissioning and delivery of emergency services at a local level and that, where a local case is made, Police and Crime Commissioners are uniquely placed to do exactly that' (2015, p.10). The UK Government is due to respond to this consultation in 2016.

The governance of the Fire and Rescue Service in England has also been the subject to a National Audit Office enquiry and one of the findings of this review was that:

> the fire and rescue service is different from other emergency services in not having an external inspectorate. The Department relies on local scrutiny (from peers within the sector, elected councilors and the general public) to safeguard service standards, governance and value for money… Councillors generally lack independent technical support and an absence of standardized information on response standards makes it hard to compare performance across different authorities (NAO 2015, p.10).

This review formed the subject of the Public Accounts House of Commons Committee meeting in November 2015 where a number of stakeholders, including officials from the Fire Officers Association, National Audit Office and Sir Ken Knight, former Chief Fire and Rescue Advisor, were there to give evidence to the Members of Parliament (PAC 2015). One of the points put to an official from the Fire Officers Association about the peer assessment whereby officers from one service monitor those of another was:

you are marking your own homework, aren't you? The police and the NHS are carefully scrutinized and there is proper oversight. Your colleagues are spending £2.1 billion of public money from council tax or direct grants, yet we have no proper independent scrutiny, no national framework for scrutiny and-I add anecdotally-a sometimes overly cosy relationship between chief fire officers, principal officers and the fire authorities (PAC p.11).

The Treasury's response to the PAC enquiry was that Fire and Rescue Services:

'governance arrangements are for local determination. Where fire and rescue services are considering a merger, or where a Police and Crime Commissioner proposes to take on responsibility for fire, the Department will work with the relevant authorities to consider the business case for change, in line with the requirements of the relevant legislation' (HM Treasury 2016). Clearly, the existing governance arrangements within the fire and rescue service is on the agenda in England.

Reviews of governance have not taken place in Wales though there has been a focus on the further enhancement of efficiency (Howell 2014), and there have been a number of framework documents outlining a need for greater scrutiny. The report of the 'Commission on Public Service Governance and Delivery' in Wales highlighted the success of the Fire and Rescue Services in Wales at reducing the number of fires and related casualties (Williams 2014). The National Issues Committee is leading on reducing costs and identifying efficiency savings. This Committee has a membership drawn from senior levels of the FRS and also a range of members of the FRA, and its role is to 'to meet the challenges facing the public sector such as economical pressures, shrinking budgets and greater public expectation...to further improve collaborative working, service delivery and sustained service improvement' (http://www.nicwalesfire.org.uk). The National Issues Committee specifically states that 'the Committee is established as a structured voluntary arrangement rather than legislatively based under the Combination Order. This demonstrates the Welsh FRA commitment to the local government model of democratically accountable by unitary authorities working close to their communities'. At a formal level, collaboration in Wales is therefore between the three Fire and Rescue Services and there are informal arrangements in place with other emergency services including shared emergency service response teams and buildings.

The national framework documents guiding the Fire and Rescue Services in Wales over a number of years have stressed key aspects around the need for FRAs to ensure local accountability and citizen inputs (Fire and Rescue National Framework 2012, 2015). The 2015 document highlights that:

members of an FRA are ultimately and collectively responsible and accountable for the decisions that it makes, and for its performance. In practice, of course, many such decisions are made by officers, who provide and seek to improve services. Nonetheless, FRA members have critical roles to play in terms of leadership and challenge. They also naturally bring an understanding of the needs and concerns of local people and communities (Fire and Rescue National Framework 2015, p.20).

The need for FRAs to engage more in the scrutiny and challenge aspects of their role was highlighted and a recommendation was made for FRAs to 'establish and maintain internal structures which clearly separate members' leadership and scrutiny roles', whilst recognising that all decisions are formally the responsibility of the authority (Fire and Rescue National Framework 2016). The governance of the FRA in Wales is an issue which the Welsh Government may consult on in the future.

Reviewing Governance

As has been highlighted above, there has been a great deal of focus within the professional literature on the need to improve governance within the Fire and Rescue Service. The existing model of governance in the Fire and Rescue Service is the stakeholder approach in which the service operates under the framework of local government with a membership drawn from locally elected members. Within this board, there is no existing academic evidence that governance is weak or that it needs to be reformed. There is, however, a lively narrative in the 'grey' literature that governance of the service needs to be improved. As highlighted in the previous section, this discussion has been going on since the 2004 Act. The shift in responsibility for the service to the Home Office in England marks a clear departure away from local government and towards central government as the 'parent'. It is clear that the narrative in England has been critical of Fire and Rescue Service governance and that the direction of travel is one of reform. This criticism has not happened to the same extent in Wales, although a different model of governance could be introduced here as well.

Taking the elements of good governance presented in this chapter, it is not clear how or whether the current stakeholder approach is failing. Clearly, if it is to be replaced, a better evidence base is needed. Are some elements of the six principles of good governance not evident enough or not in existence? Research studies of governance in practice will be required and research incorporating some observations of meetings and new data from both members of the Fire and Rescue Authority is needed. An important aspect of this will focus on the relationship between the Fire and Rescue Authority and the Fire and Rescue Service and the extent to which the authority is both leading the service and scrutinising it at the same time.

If governance is to be reformed, there are three main approaches which might be adopted and a number of variations on these. Firstly, there is the elected approach in which a directly elected commissioner or commissioners lead the service. This could be a similar structure which now exists in the police service with the Police and Crime Commissioners. The two commissioners could sit side by side or could join up to create a 'Public Protection' Officer or 'Emergency Services' Officer. This approach could bring together some of all of the different emergency services – police, ambulance and fire (www.bbc.co.uk/news/uk-29048661). To support the elected commissioners, and in order to bring in greater citizen perspective into the governance of the service, a citizen panel might be introduced. These may be similar to the police and crime panels currently in operation in the police service. This approach may go some way towards meeting one of the issues raised by Knight (2013) in his review of Fire and Rescue Service governance about the involvement of citizens. Research indicates that although these panels were intended to offer an input for citizen voice between elections, Lister and Rowe (2015, p.160) highlight that:

> PCPs offer a layer of local political accountability to the governance framework, though they do not have a direct role in holding the Chief Constable to account as that is the responsibility of PCCs themselves. It remains unclear though how robust a mechanism of 'accountability' they will provide.

A second alternative is the appointment of board members by government in new FRAs. There might be 46 of these for England and 3 for Wales or a different arrangement might be put in place. The appointment of individuals to be part of an FRA is the approach now in place in the newly formed Scottish Fire and Rescue Service with board members appointed by the Scottish Government (Scottish Government 2014). These members have replaced local authority councillors and they have been selected and appointed on the basis of the skills which they can contribute. In Scotland, the Fire and Rescue Service merged the existing eight Fire and Rescue Services in 2013 to create the national organisation, and the Scottish Government put in place a new appointment system and targets for the chair and chief officer. In their audit of the Scottish Fire and Rescue Service 1 year after the merger, the Auditor General's report (Auditor General 2015, p. 5) highlighted in relation to the new governance approach that:

> 'the board is starting to perform well and is committed to continue improving how it performs. The move away from eight local fire and rescue services to bring a national organisation has enhanced the scrutiny and challenge of the fire and rescue service'. In relation to the link with the local authorities 'the service has continued to liaise with local authorities through its network of local senior officers and through its board members'.

Devolution in the UK has brought with it the opportunity and possibility of different approaches to the governance of public services and as we have already seen in the case of the Scottish Fire and Rescue Service, a reorganised governance model which is now closer to a traditional public board in terms of the appointments to become a member, and there is also a greater focus on scrutiny and challenge (Auditor General 2015). With its new governance structure, there is the potential for greater central government control and less 'local authority' inputs as the service is now more closely managed from the centre. However, on the basis of the findings of Entwistle et al. (2015), which suggest a stronger and more positive relationship between central and local government in Scotland in comparison with other parts of the UK, greater central control through the appointment of the FRA members may not reduce local inputs in Scotland. However, this may not occur in England and Wales.

A third approach may involve elected mayors. With the changing model of governance to directly elected mayors in some areas of England, local government elected councillors have less power. Mayors are local executive leaders elected by those living within a local authority area, and they have responsibility for the whole range of public services in the area. Across England, there are elected mayors in Bristol and Manchester, for example, and with the creation of police commissioners and education commissioners in some areas, it may be that a Fire and Rescue Services commissioner is established too. All of these service commissioners could be responsible to the mayor. Alternatively, as suggested in the latest consultation document, police commissioners could take on responsibility for other emergency services including fire and rescue (HM Government 2015).

Conclusion

In any reform of the governance of the Fire and Rescue Service, a central issue in the selection of which approach to adopt is 'who owns the service?' In Scotland, the service has been taken away from local government and it is now placed more directly under central government control. The approach to reforming governance in England has not yet been decided and this is also the position in Wales. As highlighted above, there is a huge need for more research on the effectiveness of existing approaches to governance and the expected benefits of reforming this. Clearly, the agenda over a number of years, particularly in England, has been critical of the stakeholder approach and if there is a change to this model of governance, in England and Wales, then there should be valid evidence on both the need for change and the improvement in governance which will result from this.

References

Andrews, R. (2010). The impact of modernisation on fire authority performance: An empirical analysis. *Policy and Politics, 38*(4), 599–617.

Auditor General, Audit Scotland. (2015). *The Scottish fire and rescue service.* Edinburgh: Audit Scotland.

Bain, G. (2002). *Independent review of the fire service.* London: Home Office.

Brown, W. A. (2014). Antecedents to board member engagement in deliberation and decision making. In C. Cornforth & W. A. Brown (Eds.), *Nonprofit governance.* London: Routledge.

Childs, M., Morris, M., & Ingam, V. (2004). The rise and rise of clean, white-collar (fire-fighting) work. *Disaster Prevention and Management, 13*(5), 409–414.

Cornforth, C. (2003). *The governance of public and non-profit organisations: What do boards do?* London: Routledge.

DCLG. (2012). *Fire and rescue national framework for England.* London: DCLG.

De Savage, A. G. (2010). *'Localism and accountability report', fire futures.* London: DCLG.

Entwistle, T., Guarneros-Meza, V., & Martin, S. (2015). Reframing governance: Competition, fatalism and autonomy in central-local relations. *Public Administration.* doi:10.1111/padm.12210.

Farrell, C. M. (2005). Governance in the public sector: The involvement of the board. *Public Administration, 83*(1), 89–110.

Fire and Rescue National Framework. (2012). *Fire and rescue national framework, 2012 onwards.* Cardiff: Welsh Government.

Fire and Rescue National Framework. (2016). *Fire and rescue national framework 2016.* Cardiff: Welsh Government.

Fire and Rescue Services Act, 2004.

HM Government. (2015, September). *Consultation – Enabling closer working between the emergency services.* London: Home Office.

HM Treasury. (2016). *Treasury minutes – Government responses on the twenty first to the twenty sixth reports from the Committee of Public Accounts: Session 2015–16 Cm 9260*. London: Treasury.

Hood, D. (2010). *Efficiency, Effectiveness and Productivity report, Fire Futures Workstream Chair*. London: DCLG.

Howell, L. (2014). *Fire and rescue service efficiency, a report by the chief fire and rescue adviser for Wales*. Cardiff: Welsh Government.

Knight. (2013). *Facing the future – Findings from the review of effectiveness and operation in fire and rescue authorities in England*. London: Department for Communities and Local Government.

Lister, S., & Rowe, M. (2015). Elected police and crime commissioners in England and Wales: Prospecting for the democratisation of policing. *Policing and Society, 25*(4), 358–377.

Matheson, K., Manning, R., & Williams, S. (2011). From brigade to service: An examination of the role of fire and rescue services in modern local government. *Local Government Studies, 37*(4), 451–465.

McNulty, T., & Pettigrew, A. (1999). Strategists on the board. *Organization Studies, 20*(1), 47–74.

Milsted, D. (2010). *Role of the fire and rescue service (delivery models) report, fire futures*. London: DCLG.

Murphy, P., & Greenhalgh, K. (2013). Performance management in the fire and rescue services. *Public Money and Management, 33*(3), 225–232.

National Audit Office. (2015). *Financial sustainability of fire and rescue services, report by the Comptroller and Auditor General*. London: NAO.

National Issues Commission, Wales http://www.nicwalesfire.org.uk.

The F and R Service National Framework is listed in the bib as 2015.

OPM and CIPFA. (2004). *The good governance standard for public services*. London: OPM : CIPFA.

Public Accounts Committee. (2015). Oral evidence: Financial sustainability of fire and rescue services, HC582, 26th November, 2015 (Accessed on 2nd Aug 2016). https://www.nao.org.uk/wp-content/uploads/2015/11/Financial-sustainability-of-fire-and-rescue-services-amended.pdf.

Robinson, D. (2010). *Decentralisation in the Fire Sector - Empowering and Protecting the Citizen, Fire Futures, Workstream Chair*. London: DCLG.

Scottish Government. (2014). *Scottish fire and rescue service – Governance and accountability framework document*. Edinburgh: Scottish Government.

Welsh Government. (2014). *Fire and rescue service efficiency, a report by the chief fire and rescue advisor for Wales*. Cardiff: Welsh Government.

Williams, P. (2014). *Commission on public service governance and delivery*. Cardiff: Welsh Government.

www.bbc.co.uk/news/uk-29048661. (2014, September 3). Police, ambulance and fire services 'need integrating' *bbc.co.uk*.

Catherine Farrell is Professor of Public Management at the University of South Wales. Her research interests are in the areas of governance and the changing roles of professionals in public services. She has published widely on school governance and the role of public boards in public service improvement. She is currently researching different models of public board governance including the stakeholder and skills-based approaches in a range of different services including the Fire and Rescue Service, and also mapping the roles and activities of senior elite professionals in the health service. Her work has been published in journals including Public Administration, Policy and Politics, Local Government Studies, Human Relations and Industrial Relations. catherine.farrell@southwales.ac.uk

Chapter 13
Scottish Fire and Rescue Services Reform 2010–2015

Lynda Taylor, Peter Murphy, and Kirsten Greenhalgh

Introduction

Shane Ewens' excellent history of the Fire Service *Fighting Fires* (2010) shows how Scottish firefighters and Scottish services have been integral to the development of the UK Fire Service since James Braidwood established the first municipal service in Edinburgh following the great fire of 1824. Generally known as the father of firefighting, he was the first person to try to introduce a systematic method of controlling firefighting rather than simply responding and trying to cope. Braidwood transformed the perceptions and realities of urban firefighting during the industrialisation of the nineteenth century. He went on to establish the London Fire Engine Establishment in 1833, the precursor to the Metropolitan Fire Brigade of 1866. From the early nineteenth to the end of the twentieth century, there was little to differentiate the scale, scope and nature of the service in Scotland from those south of the border, as the Edinburgh 'model' has been adopted in all the great Victorian cities, such as Glasgow, Manchester, Liverpool, Birmingham, Leeds and many more.

Recent studies (Audit Scotland 2015; NAO 2015a, b; Murphy 2015a, b) have highlighted significant differences in the governance, performance and the response to the challenges of the current era of austerity in the two countries. Although the arrangements prior to 2010 were remarkably similar, since 2010, they have diverged as public sector reform, in general, and reform of the fire sector, in particular, have generated alternative policy and delivery responses, although both have embraced the move from a reactive service to a greater emphasis on prevention and protection.

L. Taylor • K. Greenhalgh
Nottingham University Business School, University of Nottingham, Nottingham, UK

P. Murphy (✉)
Nottingham Business School, Nottingham Trent University, Nottingham, UK
e-mail: Peter.Murphy@ntu.ac.uk

© Springer International Publishing AG 2018
P. Murphy, K. Greenhalgh (eds.), *Fire and Rescue Services*,
DOI 10.1007/978-3-319-62155-5_13

Nevertheless, it provides an excellent opportunity to evaluate the alternative approaches in what were previously two very similar regimes.

This chapter, therefore, explores how Scottish Fire and Rescue Services (FRSs) have evolved in the twenty-first century, after the Scottish Parliament was established in 1999 and focusses more specifically on the period 2010–2015, when the purpose, legislation, structure, objectives and performance all began to diverge from their English equivalents. Following devolution, the transfer of responsibility for fire and rescue has gradually moved from Westminster to the Scottish Executive. Although Scotland is still regulated by UK-wide legislation such as the Civil Contingencies Act (2004), the country now enacts its own legislation on the delivery of most public services, including fire and rescue (Mackie 2013).

Scotland was not subject to the Fire and Rescue Service Act of 2004, but it had its own (very similar) Fire and Rescue Services Act of 2005, to embrace the challenges of modernising the service outlined in Chapter 2. The subsequent Police and Fire Reform Act[1] (2012), however, culminated in the establishment of both a single national Fire and Rescue Service (FRS) for Scotland and a new Fire and Rescue Framework in 2013, both significantly different to their equivalents in England. The equivalent arrangements in Wales are discussed in Chapter 13.

This chapter will examine Scotland's recent approach to the structure and management of its Fire and Rescue Services. Moreover, the period from 2010 to 2015 reflects considerable changes to public service management and delivery across the UK. Despite being subject to similar funding constraints under the Coalition government's macro-economic approach to 'austerity' (Blyth 2015; O'Hara 2015; Schui 2014), Scotland has taken a very different approach to its public service design and delivery than that adopted by England. By 2015, the new governance structure in Scotland was very different to England and despite a significant transition, clear demonstrable improvement was being achieved in terms of both operational performance and efficiency savings (Audit Scotland 2015). Whilst an explicit comparison of Scotland with England is not the main aim of this chapter, the focus on Scotland, nevertheless, invites comparisons to be drawn by readers who are familiar with the English context. This chapter concludes with a brief identification of what might be some of the challenges facing the ongoing development of the single Fire and Rescue Service in Scotland.

Setting the Scene for Reform in Scottish Fire and Rescue Services

In 1973, as a result of local government reorganisation, 11 fire brigades were amalgamated into eight based on the 32 local authority areas. In 2010, the eight fire and rescue services (FRSs) had eight separate headquarter buildings with 76 whole-time fire stations, 241 retained stations and 63 volunteer stations. There were approximately 4300 whole-time firefighters, 3000 retained duty firefighters, 234 control room staff, and 1129 other support staff. The service was also assisted by 473 volunteer firefighters (Scottish Government 2011c).

The Fire Scotland Act (2005) continued the status of the services as 'local' authority services with governance overseen by Fire and Rescue Authorities (FRAs). Scottish ministers were however, given powers to further combine areas of two or more FRAs into a joint Fire and Rescue Service (Scottish Government 2011a, b, c, d). Thus, in 2010, there were two unitary fire services which covered the local authority areas of Dumfries and Galloway and Fife; and six joint fire services, which served more than one local authority area, in Grampian, Tayside, Central, Lothian and Borders, Highlands and Islands and Strathclyde.

As with the 2004 Act in England (see Chapter 3), the 2005 Act generally increased the roles and responsibilities of the Scottish services. Whilst the eight FRAs were granted more freedom to determine how resources were allocated based on local needs, this was balanced against greater responsibilities in delivering a broader role for the service, including greater emphasis on fire prevention and protection and the need to build greater national resilience against increased threats from global terrorism and extreme weather conditions. The establishment of 'Scottish Resilience', in 2008, combined the Scottish Fire Services College (the sector's national training and organisational development centre) with the Scottish Government's Fire and Civil Contingencies Division in order to strengthen Scotland's resilience to major emergencies.

Scottish minsters were also given more autonomy to determine the strategic direction of the service. A new governance structure replaced the previous statutory central advisory structure with a non-statutory arrangement through the Ministerial Advisory Group (MAG). The Fire Scotland Act (2005) expected the strategic direction of the service to be informed by a National Fire and Rescue Framework which would set out priorities, objectives and guidance for the FRAs. Between 2005 and 2010, Scottish FRSs were subject to less independent scrutiny and audit than in England. English FRS had been independently audited under the Comprehensive Area Assessment (CAA) and Comprehensive Performance Assessment (CPA) regimes, both of which published regular reports on service performance. In Scotland, under the Best Value process, there was only one independent review of the process in 2006 (Grace et al. 2007), followed by a progress review in 2007/8. The lack of regular independent performance review made it more difficult to measure progress in improvements in outcomes against the first national framework. By 2010, it was recognised that the development of more robust independent review was critical to the successful evolution of Scottish FRS (e.g. Scottish Government 2010).

In a consultation document on the future of the Fire and Rescue Service in Scotland (Scottish Government 2011), the Scottish Government set out the following vision:

> [The Scottish] Government is committed to working with stakeholders to ensure that the SFRS becomes a world class, public-focused emergency service at the heart of community resilience, with the capacity, flexibility and scale to provide 21st century fire and rescue capabilities to protect the public. (Scottish Government 2011, p. 5)

This vision was underpinned by key objectives to make Scotland *wealthier and fairer, smarter, healthier, safer and stronger and greener,* and supported by 15 national outcomes for Scotland. The consultation argued that the Scottish Fire and Rescue Service has an important role to play in the delivery of these outcomes. In particular, it contributed directly to outcome 11: *strong resilient and supportive communities, where people take responsibility for their own actions and how they affect others* and outcome 15: *public services are high quality, continually improving, efficient and responsive to local people's needs.* It is notable that the language used by the Scottish Government to describe its public services reflects a strong orientation towards ideas of 'public value', 'public governance' and 'public service' (see Benington and Moore 2014; Bovaird and Loeffler 2016; Osborne 2010; Denhardt and Denhardt 2015), whereby the users of public services are seen as citizens with responsibilities rather than from a managerial or New Public Management perspective where they are merely consumers of services. Indeed, in its key principles for fire and rescue, the consultation document stated that the service should 'demonstrate best practice in public sector governance'. As such, its key principles and vision revolved around creating a public service which was (to be) sustainable, locally responsive and accountable.[2]

Despite a clear vision, the Scottish Government recognised some key challenges faced by the service (Scottish Government 2011). These included the need to improve community fire safety and respond to increased expectations from the public. Yet, despite positive performance based on data in 2009–10,[3] fire deaths in Scotland remained high, relative to the rest of the UK. Overall deaths were 50% more likely in Scotland than England in vulnerable groups, such as people with mental health problems, a particularly high group for risk of death from fire. As in England, the 2005 Act resulted in a move away from prescriptive standards of fire cover determined centrally, towards Integrated Risk Management Planning (IRMP). Under IRMP, each service is required to prioritise its resources based on a systematic assessment of the risks to life and property in its area. The aim of IRMP is to recognise the relationship between risks and resources, and to use this information as a planning tool to ensure consistent service delivery. IRMP recognises the critical role of prevention as part of the vision for fire and rescue. Yet, despite the local focus of IRMP, a review in 2010 recommended the development of a complementary national/regional IRMP to enable economies of scale, collaboration and sharing of services such as human resources, IT and fire investigation (Scottish Fire and Rescue Advisory Unit 2010).

In order to deliver a more economic, efficient and effective FRS, the need to improve training and development, and develop wider collaboration with other blue-light services was also recognised. However, the structure of eight separate FRAs had resulted in considerable duplication of training provision. Moreover, it was argued that the ability to work collaboratively with partner agencies was potentially inhibited by the need to have eight separate but simultaneous discussions on similar areas of interest.

The unprecedented budget cuts facing Scotland (and England) only exacerbated these challenges. The coalition government's policy response to the recession led to direct cuts in public spending across the whole UK, including those available for Fire and Rescue Services. Given this financial climate, a structure of eight separate services for a relatively small country such as Scotland made significant improvements of the service appear difficult. It was also likely that under the existing structure, individual fire services would have needed to make cuts in expenditure that would have disproportionately reduced frontline services in some areas more than others. However, the Scottish Government believed the public increasingly expected consistent delivery of services, whichever area they live in.

In their manifestos for the 2011 Scottish elections, all three of the biggest parties, at that time the Scottish National Party (SNP), the Labour Party and the Liberal Democrats, acknowledged the potential benefits of a single service with the SNP and Labour the strongest advocates.

By 2011, the Scottish Government (which was now under a majority Scottish National Party Government) and the main opposition parties were individually and collectively beginning to acknowledge a potentially strong case for structural reform of the Scottish Fire and Rescue Service. Within the context of significant financial challenges and the need to provide Best Value, the Scottish government commissioned a report on the future delivery of its public services (Christie Commission 2011). This was soon followed by 'Renewing Scotland's Public Services' (Scottish Government 2011b).

The Reform of Public Services in Scotland

The Christie Commission[4] report (2011) set out the context for change in Scottish Public Services mentioned above earlier. The priorities for reform were outlined in 'Renewing Scotland's Public Services' (Scottish Government 2011b):

> The pressure on budgets is intense and public spending is not expected to return to 2010 levels in real terms for 16 years…unless Scotland embraces a radical, new collaborative culture throughout our public services, both budgets and provision will buckle under the strain. (Christie Commission 2011, p. viii)

Demographic[5] and social factors also put a strain on the demand for public services. Inequalities across Scotland accounted for a significant element of this increased demand. In general, it was estimated that up to 40% of all spending on public services was on interventions that could have been avoided by taking a more preventative approach. Focussing resources on further preventative measures in order to address these inequalities, therefore, became a key objective of reforms. Yet, it was also recognised that the organisation of public services prior to this review was plagued by systemic problems which made addressing these inequalities difficult. Services were fragmented, complex and lacking in transparency and accountability. They were also organised in a top-down way with the Scottish Government as the main arbiter and were thus unresponsive to the needs of their local communities. These problems made working with other partner agencies difficult and therefore

limited the ability of the services to deliver improved outcomes and address inequalities. The priorities for renewal of Scottish Public Services (Scottish Government
2011b) aimed to align public services with the key objectives of the Christie review.
This centred on four areas: *Prevention, Integrated Local Services, Workforce and
Leadership,* and *Improving Performance.*

Whilst the case for reform of Fire and Rescue Services had been made in the
public consultation (see above), it was not yet clear how Fire and Rescue Services
should now be structured and delivered. The case for *how* reform should happen
was put forward in an Initial Options Appraisal Report (IOAR) and further reviewed
in the Outline Business Case (OBC) (Scottish Government 2011c, d). The IOAR
included full evaluations of 14 options and was presented to the MAG at the end of
2010. The MAG agreed that further work was needed to appraise the shortlisted
options with all relevant stakeholders. Stakeholder workshops were held with
acknowledged experts. In addition, a series of visits to each separate Fire and Rescue
Service were undertaken with a view to building a comprehensive understanding of
how Fire and Rescue Services were delivered in relation to six key aspects:

- Customers
- Outcomes and products
- Processes
- People and governance
- Physical assets
- Information and technology

This information was used to further evaluate the cost, benefits, opportunities
and risks of the options shortlisted by the IOAR.

The three options for reform considered most viable,[6] included in the public
consultation on reform (Scottish Government, 2011), and fully evaluated in the
OBC, were:

- The existing eight service model but with greater collaboration encouraged and
  facilitated
- A regional model with an as yet unspecified number of regions (but commonly
  assumed to be three) to fit with wider public service reforms
- A single national Fire and Rescue Service

It was calculated that, even after accounting for the costs of transition, option
three would deliver significantly greater long-term efficiency savings[7] and greater
recurrent annual financial savings than either option one or two. Such savings could
then be reinvested to protect frontline services. Option three also scored more highly
in terms of non-monetary benefits and outcomes, including the ability of fire and
rescue to engage closely with local communities, respond quickly to future challenges and simplify its delivery mechanisms.

The potential improvement of outcomes cannot be as easily quantified as other
benefits but were, nevertheless, important. The ability of the service to improve

Table 13.1 Outcomes with examples to indicate how they might be achieved

Improved service outcomes	Examples that might illustrate success
Translation of the national outcomes into local priorities through the contribution of FRS to deliver of Single Outcome Agreements (SOA)	The delivery model should facilitate enhanced participation in the SOA processes and in local partnership working
Improving preparedness for, response to and recovery from emergencies	A standardised and more resilient approach to any emergency which occurs anywhere in Scotland, facilitating the movement of personnel, vehicles and equipment through the standardisation of equipment and procedures and a clearly defined command structure
Improving both community and firefighter safety	Standardisation of policies, procedures and partnership agreements as well as the strategic distribution of assets across Scotland to ensure adequate cover for the whole country
Ensuring appropriate and risk-based provision of fire stations, fire appliances, and crews and civil contingencies specialists to secure improved service	How the delivery model offers opportunities to ensure that an appropriate and risk-based provision of resources is maintained across Scotland to ensure adequate deployment times when they are required
Contributing to overall economic growth by mitigating the social and economic impact which fires, and other emergencies can be expected to have on individuals, commerce, industry, the environment and heritage	The delivery model offers opportunities to develop more co-ordinated and consistent approaches across Scotland to targeting groups at increased risk, through more effective education, awareness and enforcement of the delivery process

Source: Adapted from Outline Business Case (Scottish Government 2011d)

outcomes such as fire deaths was a key factor underpinning the need for reform of fire and rescue and of Scottish Public Services more generally, as discussed by the Christie Commission (2011). The most important outcome identified for FRS was the improvement of service outcomes. These are described along with examples to illustrate how they might be achieved in Table 13.1. The OBC concluded that option three had the most potential to deliver desired key outcome levels.

A single service structure would cover the whole of Scotland with a single leadership and governance structure and national approach to service delivery. National standards would help to deliver consistency in performance across Scotland. A single service structure would also enable a uniform approach to IRMP, recognised as important during its review in 2010 (see above).

Although reform towards a single service required a greater move from the status quo and was, therefore, considered a greater risk, it, nevertheless, emerged as the preferred option. Following public consultation, the decision was made to implement option three, i.e. to establish a single national Fire and Rescue Service and to provide a new Fire and Rescue Framework with objectives against which the performance of the new service could be measured.

The New Scottish Fire and Rescue Service (SFRS) and Fire and Rescue Framework

The single Scottish Fire and Rescue Service (SFRS) and Fire and Rescue Framework were both established in April 2013. The Police and Fire Reform Scotland Act (2012) provided a statutory basis for the merger of eight separate FRSs each with their own sets of executive and command staff as well as back office functions. The SFRS is now a single body which is governed and managed by a board and strategic leadership team appointed by Scottish ministers. The board provides strategic direction, support and guidance to the SFRS, ensuring that it operates effectively and that the Scottish Government's priorities are implemented. Board members are personally and corporately accountable for the board's actions and decisions. They also scrutinise plans and proposals and hold the chief officer and senior leadership team to account.

The service is organised into three Service Delivery Areas (SDAs) each with its own headquarters; one in Aberdeen (North SDA); one in Edinburgh (East SDA); and one in Hamilton (West SDA). Across the three SDAs, there are 17 local senior officers (working with clusters of co-terminus local authorities) responsible for resource management and engagement with local partners to deliver response and community safety strategies. The running of the local service areas is overseen by a deputy chief officer, responsible for corporate performance of the service. The whole of the service delivery and strategic planning is overseen and managed by a single chief officer.

Although the decision had now been made, this was recognised as only the start of a significant period of reform for Scottish Fire and Rescue. The framework for fire and rescue (Scottish Government 2013a, b) set out the strategic priorities and objectives of the new service; these priorities cover three key areas: improving service outcomes, equal access to specialist services and stronger engagement with communities. It also mirrored the shift in emphasis from property to people and from response to prevention. The intentions of each and how the service intended to meet them are summarised below.

Improving Service Outcomes and Protecting Frontline Services

The key priorities within this area cover 'risk management', 'prevention and protection', 'response and resilience' and 'the workforce'. In terms of risk management, the SFRS is responsible for reducing (fire-related) deaths in communities and mitigating the economic and social impacts of fires on those communities. As such, it needs to both identify the risks and assess them so that they can be prioritised and adequate resource can be targeted to those communities most at risk. Risk management processes and mechanisms of service delivery (prevention, protection and response) are complementary, with each informing the other. To be effective in improving outcomes, all depend heavily on planning and forming close partnerships with other agencies. For instance, the SRFS needs to maintain close links with other agencies, such as the coastguard and mountain rescue, so that its responders are provided with relevant and timely risk information. To aid in prevention, Local Senior Officers (see above) need to work with partners to identify areas most at risk, i.e. vulnerable communities, properties and the individuals that live within them.

There is an explicit emphasis on a highly skilled 'workforce' which focusses on Learning and Development. The intention is for learning and development systems to play a crucial role so that the workforce is able to learn from operational incidents and use this knowledge to improve service outcomes. The Scottish Fire Services College was to become a centre of excellence to assist in this learning and development.[8]

More Equal Access to Specialist Resources and National Capacity

In addition to fire-related duties, the SFRSs have a broader remit as set out within the 2005 Act to respond to any incident or emergency where there is a threat to life or to the environment. These other incidents or emergencies include rope and water rescue. The SFRS also provides wider services, such as rescue of people trapped in lifts, animal rescues or making buildings safe. Within the context of a single service structure, it was recognised that there should be a conscious effort to ensure that all communities have equal access to specialist services, resources and national capacity where necessary (e.g. to respond to severe weather conditions such as flooding).

Strengthened Connection Between the SFRS and Communities

The move away from eight services could have been considered risky and potentially counter-productive in light of the need for Scottish Fire and Rescue to become more responsive to the needs of local communities. Any single service would need to be underpinned by a structure that strengthened rather than weakened engagement with, and understanding of, local needs. Dedicated local senior officers were appointed by the chief fire officer (in consultation with the local authorities) to be the primary point of contact and accountable for local service delivery. Each of the 17 local senior officers has to work with their local authorities to develop priorities and objectives that reflect the needs of their local areas.

Local authorities are, therefore, now playing a key role in setting the national strategic direction of the SFRS. They also have a statutory duty to scrutinise the delivery of services in their local areas and provide feedback and recommendations on the improvement of the service to the Local Senior Officers. The 2012 Act expects local delivery of Fire and Rescue Services to become better integrated with community planning. As such, the Local Senior Officers are responsible for developing local fire and rescue plans, which must be approved by the local authority. In order to strengthen the links to local communities and become more responsive to their needs, the Local Senior Officers are responsible for describing *how* a local fire and rescue plan aims to meet locally identified priorities and outcomes.

Governance and Performance Management in the New SFRS

The new SFRS brought with it a new 'landscape' for structures of governance (Scottish Government, 2013). New governance and accountability arrangements are set out in the 'Governance and Accountability Framework Document' (Scottish Government 2013a). Public sector governance arrangements generally involve accountability mechanisms relative to the stated goals of the sector, e.g. effective service outcomes as in the case of the SFRS. It also usually includes the structures that clarify the responsibilities of the various stakeholders to the organisation, and the tools that could be used to assure accountability both internally and externally (Annisette et al. 2013). National and local democratic accountabilities are the dominant mechanisms by which those in authority are held to account for the effective running of the SFRS. The new accountability framework includes the roles and responsibilities of ministers, Scottish Government, the SFRS chair, board and chief officer.

Roles and responsibilities demand good conduct from those in authority in order to meet the stated objectives of the SFRS. For instance, the chief officer must ensure *…robust performance and risk management arrangements…to support the achievement of the SFRS's aims and objectives and that facilitate comprehensive reporting to the board, the Scottish Government and the wider public* (Scottish Government 2013a, p. 6). Comprehensive reporting refers to transparency, which is also a key mechanism for ensuring effective governance by providing the openness needed to, amongst other things, prevent the abuse of power (Bovens et al. 2014). The SFRS has a statutory duty to provide the public as well as national and local government with access to its proceedings, papers and reports.

Audit and scrutiny arrangements provide the tools needed to assure the accountability of the SFRS both internally for the purposes of internal control (to prevent fraud and theft) and externally for its stakeholders including the Scottish Government and wider public. The Auditor General for Scotland (Audit Scotland) has the powers to examine value for money and financial performance. In addition, Her Majesty's Chief Fire Service Inspector in Scotland (HMCFSIS) oversees operational inspection of the SFRS, including community safety engagement, staff learning and development, and policies and practices. Both bodies, i.e. HM Fire Service Inspectorate in Scotland (HMFSI) and Audit Scotland have a duty to undertake complementary scrutiny activity covering areas such as outcomes, service performance, partnership working and community planning. In practice, they liaise closely and operate collaboratively. Since 2010, Scotland has strengthened independent scrutiny of its FRS. In contrast, in England, unlike Scotland, governance and performance management of the English Fire and Rescue Service has been more influenced by notions of localism and sector-led improvement with a greater emphasis on 'New Public Management', particularly since the coalition government came to power in 2010 (DCLG 2012; LGA 2011, LGA 2014, Lowndes and Pratchett 2012, Downe et al. 2014; Murphy and Greenhalgh 2014; Murphy and Jones 2016).

Arguably, the ultimate aim of effective governance is to help organisations achieve their objectives. Performance information can help with effective internal control and inform external stakeholders about how well the organisation is doing (Annisette et al. 2013). Performance management regimes based upon notions of 'Public Value' would expect those responsible for service delivery to develop publicly accountable measures which demonstrate that objectives have been achieved and would emphasis public involvement (Moore 1995; Benington and Moore 2014). As such, the Scottish Government and the SFRS's independent board define specific performance targets, and the system uses independent audit and scrutiny arrangements to hold the SFRS accountable for their achievement. Scottish ministers hold the SFRS to account for performance against key targets. As detailed within the Fire and Rescue Framework and the SFRS's Planning and Performance Management Framework (SFRS 2014), these targets are:

- Reducing fire fatalities and causalities
- Reducing special service fatalities and casualties
- Reducing accidental dwelling fires
- Reducing the number of non-domestic fires
- Reducing firefighter injuries
- Reducing staff sickness absence

The aim of the targets is to assess the realisation of reform benefits but also provide a basis for continuous improvement of the service. It is recognised that not all targets would be applicable at the local level, and targets may need to be adapted to suit local risk profiles. The Planning and Performance Management Framework developed by the SFRS in 2014 builds on the Fire and Rescue Framework to show how the SFRS plans to achieve the relevant targets. For instance, the document contains a high-level strategy map to show the performance indicators which underpin the achievement of the high-level targets and how the targets map to outcomes and the SFRS's strategic aims.

Conclusions

Within the broader context of public service management and delivery, this chapter has sought to understand how and why Scottish Fire and Rescue Services have evolved and changed since devolution. In particular, this chapter has emphasised reform of the Scottish Fire and Rescue Services from eight separate services to a single service structure. The reasons for such reform were not unique to Scotland but indicative of a range of similar internal and external factors also experienced by other countries. For instance, most OECD countries (and many others) have experienced recession since 2008, producing falling tax revenues, increasing welfare payments and rising fiscal deficits (Bovaird and Loeffler 2016). Cutting the cost of public services (rather than increasing taxes) has been adopted as the most appropriate response by many countries, including the UK.

Nevertheless, despite the financial (and other) pressures faced by Scotland (which have been similar to the rest of the UK) the answer has not been a further entrenchment of 'New Public Management' philosophy, e.g. through the use of internal market mechanisms; often couched within the language of 'choice'. Rather, in Scotland, the aim has been to maintain a more 'public interest/public value' ethos behind the delivery of its public services; one that is built on reducing inequalities and generally aiming to improve the social and economic aspects of the lives of those in local communities. Notably, it is not assumed, that creating competition (through means of private sector involvement) is a more efficient way of doing so. The priority for reform of fire and rescue has been based around a philosophy that aims to deliver an improved service by reducing the duplication of services that could be shared as an alternative to cutting frontline services, which they argued would have made inequalities even worse in some communities. In conclusion, although there were evident financial constraints, the *way* in which Scotland has chosen to reform its Fire and Rescue Service was based around notions of creating 'public value' and the delivery of an economic, efficient and effective service within a central ethos of fairness and equality across Scotland.

Democratic accountability is a key feature of Scottish Public Services. As such, in the SFRS, governance mechanisms have been improved in order to strengthen (rather than weaken) public assurance. In addition to the government itself and the Board, Audit Scotland[9] and HMSSI[10] provide strengthened independent scrutiny and oversight of the service against the 2013 Fire and Rescue Framework,[11] including the performance targets outlined earlier.

In May 2015, Audit Scotland (2015) concluded that 'the Scottish Government and the SFRS had managed the 2013 merger of the eight legacy services effectively – the reform of Scottish Fire and Rescue through creation of the SFRS had no detrimental impact on the public, and its performance was improving. The move from eight local Fire and Rescue Services to a national organisation had enhanced the scrutiny and challenge of the Fire and Rescue Service. Reported savings to date puts the Scottish Fire and Rescue Service on track to exceed expected savings of £328 million by 2027/28'. (2015, p. 5).

Scotland, at least in terms of its fire and rescue service, had witnessed a successful transformation project that demonstrated individual and collective leadership and a strategic and holistic approach to the service. It led to more robust governance and scrutiny arrangements and improved service outcomes. During the same period, England saw an abdication of leadership responsibilities, particularly from the DCLG, minimal and ad hoc restructuring resulting in loss of public accountability, suboptimal delivery and significant risks to the achievement of Value for Money (NAO 2015a, b; Murphy 2015a, b).

During the time period covered in this chapter, the nature, purpose and organisational structure of the service have changed. However, SFRS had not yet addressed reform of the services' operational stations which were scheduled for a later phase of reform. At the time of writing this chapter, the UK macro-economic policy which involves restricting resources to the public sector has been reconfirmed in a further 3-year spending review. The outcome of the EU referendum has led us into a further period of economic turmoil and uncertainty. Moreover, in the Scottish elections of 2016, the SNP lost their overall majority and emerged as a minority government.

Notes

1. Although the legislative framework and timetable have been similar for fire service and the new police services, implementation of reform in the police has proven far more problematical than in the fire service to date.
2. Sir Peter Housden the former permanent secretary of the ODPM and Department of Communities and Local Government (2005–2010) was permanent secretary of the Scottish Government from June 2010 to June 2015.
3. 2009–10 data indicate a general decline in the number of all types of fires in Scotland, with rates down by a third across both primary and secondary fires. Dwelling fires – where most fire fatalities occur – have shown a continuing decline, reflecting the focus on prevention activities. The figures for dwelling fires show a decrease of 30% since 1999 (Scottish government 2011d).
4. The make-up and conduct of the Christie Commission was very much in the spirit of former Royal Commissions of the past.
5. Projections suggested that the population of Scotland will rise from 5.19 million (as of June 2009) to 5.54 million by 2033. It will also age significantly, with the numbers of people aged 60 and over increasing by 50% from 1.17 m to 1.75 m. This, combined with the trend towards increasing numbers of elderly and single-occupancy households, will increase dwelling fire risk'. (Scottish Government 2011d, p. 28).
6. In the run-up to the 2015 general election, the Shadow Fire Minister Lyn Brown MP issued a consultation on proposed structural changes to the fire services in England. This had three options: voluntary local mergers, a new regional structure based on the nine English regions and a single national service. When the Conservatives won the election, they preferred to bring forward proposals to allow police and crime commissioners to take responsibility for Fire and Rescue Services.
7. Valued at £293 m over 15 years compared with £215 m for option 2. (Scottish Government 2011d).
8. In England both the Fire Service College in Gloucestershire and the Emergency Planning College at Easingwold have been sold to private sector contractors.

9. Since 2000, shortly after devolution, Audit Scotland has been responsible for auditing both central and local government as well as the NHS in Scotland. In England, these were previously divided between the Audit Commission and the National Audit Office.
10. Unlike the Chief Fire and Rescue Advisor in England (who is a departmental civil servant), HMFSI in Scotland is independent of the government.
11. At the time of writing, a new Fire and Rescue Framework for 2016 is under public consultation.

References

Annisette, M., Cooper, C., & Neu, D. (2013). Public sector governance and accountability. *Critical Perspectives on Accounting, 24*, 479–487.
Audit Scotland. (2015). *Scottish fire and rescue service*. Edinburgh: Audit Scotland.
Benington, J., & Moore, M. (Eds.). (2014). *The theory and practice of public value*. Basingstoke: Palgrave Macmillan.
Blyth, M. (2015). *Austerity: The history of a dangerous idea*. Oxford: Oxford University Press.
Bovaird, T., & Loeffler, E. (2016). *Public management and governance* (3rd ed.). London, New York: Routledge.
Bovens, M., Goodin, R. E., & Schillemans, T. (2014). *The oxford handbook of public accountability*. Oxford: Oxford University Press.
Christie Commission. (2011). *Report of the commission on the future delivery of public services*. Edinburgh: The Scottish Government.
Denhardt, J. V., & Denhardt, R. B. (2015). *The new public service: Serving, not steering* (4th ed.). New York: Routledge.
Department of Communities and Local Government. (2012). *National framework for fire and rescue authorities in England*. London: HMSO.
Downe, J., Martin, S., & Doring, H. (2014). *Evaluation of the operational assessment and fire peer challenge programme*. London: LGA/CFOA.
Ewen, S. (2010). *Fighting fires: Creating the British fire service 1800–1978*. Basingstoke: Palgrave macmillan.
Grace, C., Nutley, S., Downe, J., & Martin, S. (2007). *Decisive moment: Report of independent review of the best value audit process*. Edinburgh: Audit Scotland.
Local Government Association. (2011). *Taking the lead: Self-regulation and improvement in local government*. London: LGA.
Local Government Association. (2014). *Evaluation of sector-led improvement*. London: LGA.
Lowndes, V., & Pratchett, L. (2012). Local governance under the coalition government: Austerity, localism and the big society. *Local Government Studies, 38*(1), 21–40.
Mackie, R. (2013). *Managing Scotland's public services*. Edinburgh: Sweet and Maxwell.
Moore, M. H. (1995). *Creating public value*. Cambridge, MA: Harvard Business University Press.
Murphy, P. (2015a). *Briefing note on 'Financial sustainability of fire and rescue services – value for money report' for the National Audit Office*. Nottingham: NTU.
Murphy, P. (2015b). *Briefing note on the 'Impact of funding reductions on fire and rescue services': Local government report for the National Audit Office*. Nottingham: NTU.
Murphy, P., & Greenhalgh, K. (2014). Peer challenge needs an independent fire inspectorate. *FIRE, 110*, 17–19.
Murphy, P., & Jones, M. (2016). Building the next model for intervention and turnaround in poorly performing local authorities in England. *Local Government Studies, 42*(5), 698–716.

National Audit Office. (2015a). *Financial sustainability of fire and rescue services value for money report*. London: NAO.

National Audit Office. (2015b). *Financial sustainability of fire and rescue services local government report*. London: NAO.

O'Hara, M. (2015). *Austerity bites: A journey to the sharp end of the cuts in the UK*. Bristol: Policy Press.

Osborne, S. P. (2010). *The new public governance*. London, New York: Routledge.

Schui, F. (2014). *Austerity: The great failure*. New Haven: Yale University Press.

Scottish Fire and Rescue Advisory Unit. (2010). *Review of the implementation and impact of integrated risk management planning in Scottish fire and rescue services*. Edinburgh: Scottish Government.

Scottish Government. (2010). *Commission on Public Services. Firts Minister Alex Salmond tatement on the Launch of the Christie Commission. 19th November 2010*. Edinburgh: Scottish Government.

Scottish Fire and Rescue Service. (2014). *Planning and performance management framework*. Edinburgh: SFRS.

Scottish Government. (2011a). *A consultation on the future of the fire and rescue service in Scotland*. Edinburgh: Scottish Government.

Scottish Government. (2011b). *Renewing Scotland's public services*. Edinburgh: Scottish Government.

Scottish Government. (2011c). *Initial options appraisal report: Prepared for Scottish fire and rescue services ministerial advisory group*. Edinburgh: Scottish Government.

Scottish Government. (2011d). *Reform of the fire and rescue service in Scotland: outline business case*. Edinburgh: Scottish Government.

Scottish Government. (2013a). *Fire and rescue framework for Scotland*. Edinburgh: Scottish Government.

Scottish Government. (2013b). *Scottish fire and rescue service (SFRS) governance and accountability framework*. Edinburgh: Scottish Government.

Dr. Lynda Taylor Following completion of her Ph.D. at the University of Manchester, Lynda joined Nottingham University Business School as an Assistant Professor of Accounting in 2006. Lynda publishes her research mainly within high-quality management accounting journals. Her interests include performance measurement, risk management and qualitative accounting research. More recently, Lynda's interests have expanded into public management and, in particular, accountability and performance within the public sector. Since 2015, she has been collaborating on a project about accountability within the UK Fire and Rescue service, specifically comparing the diverging performance management and accountability regimes of England and Scotland from 2010 to 2016.

Chapter 14
Command and Control of Fire and Rescue Operations in Sweden

Stefan Svensson

Introduction

Before the mid-1800s, when a fire occurred, it was a local matter to organise the efforts to control the fire, and it was in the interest of everyone within that community to assist in these efforts. However, the efforts were not always efficient, and the education and training in fire suppression was non-existent. After a large number of severe fires, where large parts of a number of cities were burned to the ground, the first national fire code was issued in 1873 (Räddningsverket 1992). During this period, the first fire brigades were organised and officers were recruited from the military simply because they were known to have the ability to organise manpower and equipment (Michal 1993).

As a consequence, the fire brigades were organised in a, for that period, typical military style including their education and training. The focus was on discipline, giving orders and uniforms. At about the same time, new technology was introduced and motor vehicles, including pumps and ladders, became increasingly used even in the fire service.

Education and training of fire officers as well as the manpower was to a very large extent based on experience, and out of this a system of apprentices–masters grew. It should be noted that knowledge on fire behaviour, properties of materials subjected to fire as well as efficient commanding systems was very low at this point. Experience was considered to be the key to success, which is something we can still see in the fire and rescue service today, for good and bad.

Although there were early attempts to create practical guides based on the level of knowledge of that time (see, e.g. Shaw 1876), it was not until the mid-1900s that more scientific approaches to the work undertaken by the fire and rescue service can be found. Fire suppression was one of these early subjects for research, including

S. Svensson (✉)
Division of Fire Safety Engineering, Lund University, Lund, Sweden
e-mail: stefan.svensson@brand.lth.se

© Springer International Publishing AG 2018   207
P. Murphy, K. Greenhalgh (eds.), *Fire and Rescue Services*,
DOI 10.1007/978-3-319-62155-5_14

the work by, for example, Clark (1947), Hird et al. (1954), Thomas and Smart (1954), Simms and Hinkley (1959) and Thomas (1959). A large number of the conclusions from this early research are still valid and apply very well in the modern fire and rescue service community. But, it was not until very recently that a more scientific view on the fire and rescue service can be seen. Of course, this includes problems related to command and control.

Regulations aimed at the fire and rescue service have evolved over the years and one of the major changes was made in the Fire Law issued in 1974. Here, the formal responsibility to deal with not only fires but more or less every type of accident was given to the fire and rescue services. In practice, this was already the case, but it had to be regulated which also led to consequences relating to command and control.

Today, the fire and rescue service deals with a large variety of accidents and the command system must be such that it can be adapted to accidents of different characteristics, types and sizes. And, as in many other countries, the personnel involved in providing the service are to a large extent part time (similar to paid volunteers) which puts even further demands on simple but functional command systems.

Regulating the Fire and Rescue Service: Local Self-Government and Cooperation

An important basis for the Swedish parliamentarianism is local self-government, which means that local authorities are responsible for local or regional issues and they have a very wide discretion (Local government act 1991:900). In short, the government does not generally interfere with local matters. This local self-government has deep historical roots, and it aims to give people responsibility and influence over common and local issues. Autonomy is exercised by decision-making bodies appointed by universal suffrage and representing local people. Municipalities are the local self-government bodies, and they have the right to levy taxes by citizens to finance their operations, including the fire and rescue service.

In Sweden, there are 290 municipalities and 20 counties. Their responsibilities include local issues such as infrastructure, housing and business development, and welfare services such as schools, elderly care and health care. The mission of the municipalities has, since 1862, been to manage its 'internal matters of common concern' and developing and operating a well-functioning society at local and regional level, with citizen participation and accountability of elected representatives. The county council share health and to some extent traffic and business development.

Consequently, local self-government has an impact on activities by the fire and rescue services. Municipalities are responsible for service within their geographical area, and they may organise the fire service more or less as they please. However, there are safety regulations as well as a few general requirements they have to fulfil (Civil protection act 2003:778; Civil protection regulation 2003:789; AFS 2007:7).

This includes responsibility to have an organisation with ability to respond to accidents and incidents, and requirements on responsibilities for incident commanders. But, and this is an important aspect of local self-government, there are not really any regulations or requirements on staffing, response time and equipment (apart from more general safety aspects). Each and every municipality may organise and equip their fire and rescue service as they please, although the impact through training, inter-municipal cooperation, history and traditions is large. Therefore, there are more similarities than differences as a nation overall when it comes to how the fire service works at accident sites.

The consequence of this lack of regulations is that it can lead to a large variation in the preparedness (numbers of firefighters and response time), which is not necessary in proportion to the population size. So, for example, in the most southern fire and rescue organisation, there is an overall preparedness of 60 firefighters and fire officers located in 12 fire stations (Räddningstjänsten Syd 2011). This covers a population of approximately 513,000 inhabitants (www.scb.se), which gives a ratio of about 8500 inhabitants per firefighter. At a fire and rescue organisation on the northern coast, there is a total number of 41 firefighters and fire officers in preparedness (Engström 2011). The population is approximately 63,000 inhabitants (www.scb. se). This gives a ratio of about 1500 inhabitants per firefighter. On the other hand, the population density in the area covered by the southern organisation is approximately 670 inhabitants per square kilometre. The population density in the area covered by the northern organisation is approximately 13 inhabitants per square kilometre (www.scb.se). Consequently, getting a reasonable response time in a less densely populated area requires a larger number of firefighters, relatively speaking.

Responding to incidents and accidents is based on cooperation between several authorities. From a strict legal point of view, each actor (mainly including the fire and rescue service, the police and the emergency medical service) have a rather well-defined remit, although there are common areas of interest. It should be noted that the fire and rescue service is a local responsibility, the emergency medical service is a responsibility for the county (regional) and the police is a national organisation. Each authority has staff trained to meet the organisation's mission (again, from a legal point of view). No organisation has the right to give directives over the others, which is a consequence of the local self-government system. But, in most cases, it requires several different skills to assess an event and act so that the public's need for assistance is handled effectively. Therefore, responding actors identify the need for assistance together and design their various actions as a whole (Fredholm and Göransson 2006). One can say that the responding agencies set the scene for each other. However, it requires each operator to be able to see the situation from a holistic perspective. Consequently, situations requiring flexibility, foresight, quick decisions and fast action can be difficult to handle, especially when several authorities are involved.

The Swedish overall emergency preparedness is based on society's normal, daily activities to prevent and handle accidents and less extensive disorders. In the case of serious incidents or crises in society, these resources can be strengthened. Emergency preparedness is thus the capacity created in many actors' daily business and not a designated organisation or an actor (www.msb.se). Basic principles in the emergency preparedness are:

- Responsibility – an organisation that has responsibility for operations in normal situations also has a similar responsibility during a crisis or societal disruption. Actors affected by such an event, direct or indirect, that can help to deal with consequences also have a responsibility to act during a crisis. Consequently, actors should support and cooperate with each other.
- Proximity – that social disorders should be managed where they occur,
- by those who are most affected and responsible, at as low a hierarchical level as possible.
- Equality – actors should not make major changes in their organisation other than needs inflicted by the event. Operations during major events will function as during normal conditions, as far as possible.
- Geographical area – responsibility to ensure coordination between all those involved in emergency preparedness at local, regional and central level. Municipalities have the geographical area of responsibility within their geographical area, county councils within the geographical area of the county and government for the entire country.
- Sector accountability – the responsibility of government authorities for their issues of national importance, regardless of geographic extension.

However, these basic principles have been questioned in recent years. Consequently, they might change in the future although it would require a lot of time and effort to do so.

In the case of an extraordinary event, defined as, 'an event that deviates from the norm, implies a serious disturbance or imminent risk of a serious disturbance in important societal functions and requires urgent action by a municipality or a county council, a crisis management committee should be established' (2006:544), such a committee may decide to take over all or part of the areas of activity from other committees in the municipality or county council to the extent that is necessary in view of the extraordinary event's type and scope. An extraordinary event may impact upon resource availability. As resources become limited, there may be a requirement for a more thorough assessment decision about which type of incidents (based on size, characteristics, geographical area, etc.) should be responded to. However, the functions of the fire and rescue service remain although a crisis management committee can decide upon such matters.

Responsibilities and Regulations

Society has a responsibility to prevent accidents as well as to provide help when accidents do occur. The municipalities are one of the organisations which are responsible when there are accidents or there is imminent danger of accidents occurring, to prevent or limit damage to people, property or the environment, within their respective geographical area. The inter-municipal organisation primarily responsible for this on a daily basis is denoted and known as the fire and rescue services.

The fire and rescue service in Sweden is primarily regulated by the Civil Protection Act (2003:778) and in the civil protection regulation (2003:789) concerning the protection against accidents. The legislation includes provisions for individuals, municipalities and the county, and it is designed to provide reasonable protection against accidents to people, property and the environment throughout the country, taking into account local conditions. The Civil Protection Act is a framework, which means that it, to a greater extent, includes basic values and principles and, to a lesser extent, details what should be done and how this will be accomplished, in agreement with the local self-governing system. The national government cannot make any decisions upon the level of protection locally.

According to this legislation, everyone across the country is entitled to some level of protection against accidents, but the actual level of ambition and how the service is provided, organised and implemented may look different depending on where you reside. It is a local decision made by local politicians. It may, therefore, differ between municipalities, or even within the same municipality, which equipment is alerted, which methodology is used or how much staff is dispatched to an accident. Note, however, that although there are no design rules, or equivalent, the differences between municipalities are generally very small. What can really differ is partly access to technical equipment, staffing, and terms and concepts. Due to the educational system, similarities are very large, although there may still be differences over the country, in terms of quantity as well as quality and tactics.

The responsibilities by local and national authorities are to respond to accidents or imminent danger of accidents to prevent or limit damage to people, property or the environment (2003:778). The law draws a distinction between national and municipal rescue services. National emergency service covers mountain rescue, search for missing persons, environmental rescue at sea, aircraft search and rescue, and the response to the release of radioactive substances. Any other emergency services (except medical emergencies) are local, provided for by the municipals (i.e. the fire and rescue service).

One should also keep in mind that both national and municipal rescue services can be at the same event at the same time. There may even be several different national and municipal organisations, each responsible for their operation, respectively, at the same accident/event. Consequently, cooperation and collaboration is a prerequisite for an effective response, but it is particularly important when several different types of organisations are involved. An example of this can be if an aircraft goes missing, that is, if it disappears from the radar screen at the air traffic control. Such a situation can be complex, since the Civil Aviation Authority is responsible for air rescue (according to Civil Protection Regulation 2003:789 and Aviation Regulation 1986:171) when an aircraft is in distress or when danger threatens air traffic. However, if the crash site is (or is expected to be) in the large lakes of Sweden (Vänern, Vättern and Mälaren) or in Swedish territorial waters and exclusive economic zone, the JRCC (Joint Rescue Coordination Centre) is responsible for actions. At a crash site in the mountain area, the police force is responsible for a rescue operation, and if the crash site is on land, including other lakes than Vänern, Vättern and Mälaren, such as waterways, canals and municipal harbour areas, the municipal fire and rescue service is responsible. But, as long as the crash site is not known, each of these organisations may initiate a response since there is a high probability that an incident may arise. On top of this, the emergency medical service (which is a regional/county responsibility) might initiate a response. Consequently, there can be several rescue operations initiated from different actors (local, regional and national) at the same time and to the same (expected) event. When the crash site is known, each of the actors has their respective resources that may be needed for an effective response. Depending on the actual crash site, the resources used may differ. The need for cooperation is, therefore, large (Räddningsverket 2008).

Accidents and Operations

The fire and rescue service is expected to respond to basically any type of accident or incident, ranging from fires to car accidents, medical calls, flooding and even the classic cat-in-a-tree (although this last example may not be an operation from a strict legal point of view). The reason for this is most likely traditional along with the availability of tools, techniques and knowledge. It is also likely to be connected to the strong local presence: in smaller villages, everyone knows a fireman and the firemen know their locals.

A fire and rescue operation is the term normally used for the phenomenon in which all or part of the municipal emergency organisation, that is, the fire and rescue service, is dispatched to an accident, with the task to put things right, that is, to help those who are in need. Such an operation can be defined as a phenomenon in which one or more actions are initiated, coordinated and implemented under the management of one or more commanding officers, in order to offer assistance in case of accident or imminent danger of an accident. Such operations are often carried out in a dynamic environment, and the operation shall include an incident commander (Svensson et al. 2009).

In order not to jeopardise the effectiveness of the emergency services, the responsibility to intervene may be limited. The municipality is only obliged to intervene and conduct fire and rescue operations if this is justified by (Civil Protection Act 2003:778):

- The need for rapid intervention
- The threatened interests
- Costs of the operation
- Other circumstances

Each of these criteria must be met for the municipality to be obliged to intervene. Similarly, the operation shall be terminated when one or more of these criteria are no longer met. In practice, it may, in some cases, be difficult to assess when it is justified for a municipality to be responsible for the services. Above all, it can be difficult to assess when the emergency situation is over and the operation can be terminated. However, the fire and rescue service can still respond to an event although it is not a rescue operation according to the criteria above. What the municipalities do with their resources, apart from rescue operations according to the Civil Protection Act, is a local decision.

From a practical perspective, it is not always easy to define an accident and to what extent society (the municipality) should help individuals and organisations in distress. Apart from legal requirements, the historical development has led to a view in which it is considered reasonable for the fire and rescue service to fight a fire but also to avert and limit other hazards, injuries or accidents such as road accidents or accidents involving hazardous chemicals. But it is not always obvious when the fire and rescue service is required to intervene.

For larger events, or events of a catastrophic nature, it can be difficult to determine if the event generates one or more emergency responses. Factors that may affect the assessment include (Svensson et al. 2009):

- Physical perspective on the accident

  - Object
  - Size, type, natural boundaries, etc.
  - Propagation
  - Size of the accident
  - Cause–effect

- Resources

  - Competition over limited resource, that is, resources that limit what can be performed or accomplished

- Organisation/Management

  - Organisational synergies with common management
  - Practical – organisational (logistics, transportation, etc.)
  - Closeness in geography
  - Ability to monitor input/actions
  - Collaboration with other organisations.

How an operation is defined should be based on the option that is most beneficial based on the factors above. A problem here is that one seldom assesses and defines an operation other than when the question relates to financial compensation. Many times, one should also consider and define operations from a managerial, practical or physical perspective (ibid).

The basis for an operation leading to an intervention by the fire and rescue service is that a need for help has occurred due to an accident – someone is in distress, someone who cannot handle the situation and therefore is in the need for assistance. The idea of initiating a response fails without this need for assistance. Thus, there is no end in itself to carry out fire and rescue operations. We also have to put the concept of an operation in the context of a disaster: one can thus say that the need for help in such cases locally in time or space exceeds the ability of society to cope with this need with its own resources (Svensson et al. 2009). The question of cooperation and collaboration is central, and there may be reasons to use organisations and resources that are not normally used during accidents and incidents. Examples of such organisations may be ecclesial communities, armed forces or other municipal administrations than the fire service such as social services, environmental agencies or technical departments. It may also be agencies that are not normally associated with emergency services, such as the National Veterinary Institute, National Food Administration, Swedish Transport Administration, the Swedish Board of Agriculture or even the Swedish Tax Agency.

Organising the Fire and Rescue Service

As mentioned above, there are no national design rules (or similar) for the fire and rescue service, with a few very specific exceptions related to safety. Each municipality is free to develop their own guidelines, to set their own targets for their operations and to design and organise them in the way they best see fit, depending on local circumstances.

One of the exceptions is related to traffic accidents. Through training, certain common practices have been developed which largely focus on the patient and where cooperation with emergency medical service is in focus (Wargclou 2010; Räddningsverket 2008). Similarly, based on regulations for interior firefighting issued by the Work Environment Authority, a common basis for actions in cases of fire in buildings has been developed over a long period of time. These regulations stipulate that interior firefighting with the use of breathing apparatus requires a minimum of five firefighters (two on the inside, one in the door, a pump operator and an officer). Consequently, many fire crews are based on this, so a crew of five is very common. Safety to firefighting personnel is placed very highly. However, there are a large number of safety aspects to consider during fire and rescue operations, some of which are regulated through the Work Environment Authority (www.av.se).

A fire and rescue service organisation is mainly based on line organisations and a hierarchical approach to management, although the work at an accident site, in many cases, requires a high degree of flexibility. In a line organisation, authority flows from top to bottom and accountability goes upwards from the bottom along the chain of command. In some cases, management is supported by a staff, and one can speak of a line-staff organisation. In such an organisation, emphasis is on the team's overall specialist role, the staff provides data for the manager's decision and the team consists of experts available at the department's disposal. In most Swedish fire and rescue organisations, the command system is very flexible, and ranks are rarely used in terms of claiming authority over others. An officer is, in many cases, considered to be a member of the team.

Traditionally, the fire and rescue service has been organised on the basis of training and qualifications achieved through training: members of the organisation have ranks based on their training qualifications. As was mentioned earlier, there is a fairly strong military tradition.

In most cases, the fire service is organised in three or four command levels. A crew commander, which is the first level, is in charge of two to seven firefighters. A station officer (on-scene commander), which is the second level of command, is in charge of two to four crew commanders and a chief officer (incident commander) is in charge of two to four station officers. However, even a very large event, such as a fire in a large industrial facility, requirement rarely exceeds more than 40–60 firefighters, but this is more than most municipalities have available themselves. Also, it should be noted that the head officer of the organisation (a fire chief or a commissioner) has overall responsibility and may at any time assume command over an operation. This rarely happens, but it gives this head officer the possibility to decide upon allocation of resources between two (or more) simultaneously ongoing operations, replace incident commanders or decide long-term objectives for complex or time-consuming operations.

Also, there is an increasing attention paid to expertise in a different way than before, and different types of general management roles have been introduced. The purpose of this is primarily to be able to manage the operation more effectively and to allocate resources in time or space at several simultaneous operations or during disasters. Through such a more modern view on officers, the attention has also increasingly become focussed on skills, abilities and not least suitability. In most cases people in the fire service climb in ranks based on their competency, and not on degrees or years of experience, as may have been the case in previous years.

Incident Commanders

An incident commander plays a special role at operations and some very specific obligations and responsibilities are related to this role. According to Swedish Law (2003:778), there must be an incident commander at any fire and rescue operation. Only fire officers can be incident commanders, and their qualifications are regulated by law. The purpose of having an appointed (and competent) incident commander is, of course, to effectively and safely carry out and manage operations. Depending on the type, characteristics and nature of an incident, the role of the incident commander can be carried out by a fire chief, but it is usually assigned to a station officer or a crew commander, depending on the type and characteristics of an incident. However, each municipality may organise this in any way they please, as long as the qualifications for competency are fulfilled (as required by national regulations, 2003:789, due to the obligations and responsibilities linked to the incident commander).

Since the obligations and responsibilities that come with the role of incident commander involve restrictions on civil rights and liberties, these must be addressed consistently and based on informed judgements. These obligations and responsibilities include (2003:778):

- To initiate and end fire and rescue operations
- Interference with the rights of others
- Impose a duty on civilians to serve
- Conduct surveillance at the expense of others
- Request assistance of other authority
- Notify the authority responsible for defects or irregularities that could lead to other emergencies

Incident commanders must, of course, not make decisions on these issues arbitrarily or by tradition: each decision must be substantiated and assessed against a specific situation. The decision must be necessary and the action or actions leading to the decision must outweigh the intrusion on the individual or individuals affected by the decision. The obligations and responsibilities, therefore, put fairly high demands on the skills of the individual who is the incident commander.

Decisions made regarding these obligations and responsibilities must be reported in writing. The decision must specify when and by whom the decision is taken, the reasons for the decision and to whom it relates. If the incident commander is not at the scene in person, which is fully legitimate, for example, at a command centre, there are high demands on good, thoughtful and informed decision-making including effective and clear communication between the incident commander and on-scene commanders.

Initiate and End Fire and Rescue Operations

The incident commander decides when a rescue operation is to be ended, a decision that must be reported in writing. When the operation comes to an end, the incident commander or the on-scene commander should also, if possible, notify the owner or tenant of the property that the operation has been ended and of the need for security, salvage, restoration and recovery. In many cases, a so-called salvage officer is called to the scene, which is based on an agreement between insurance companies and the municipalities. This salvage officer has the right to take measures needed to save as much property as possible, from an economical point of view.

It should also be noted that the initiation of an operation is a formal decision as well. However, this initiation is in most cases based upon more vague grounds, since the municipality has a general duty to carry out fire and rescue operations when the need arises. Consequently, the municipality also has a duty to examine the facts when it receives information or indication about events that can possibly lead to a fire and rescue operation (or some other type of response) (MSBFS 2012:5).

Interference with the Rights of Others

The incident commander may decide to interfere with the rights of others. This means that the incident commander in a rescue operation may gain themselves and their staff access to others' property (other than that involved in the operation, such as a neighbour) cordoning off or evacuating areas, use, remove or destroy property, and make other interventions in the rights of others, to the extent that the procedure is justified with respect to the nature of the danger, the injury caused and other circumstances. It may also include placing of devices needed for the operation on someone else's land or in a building. Decisions on interference with rights of others imply that there is danger to life, health or property, or harm to the environment, and this cannot be prevented in any other way. The police are obliged to provide the necessary assistance when such decisions are made.

Request of Duty by Civilians to Serve

The incident commander may impose duties on civilians to serve. This means that the person who is of an age between 18 and 65 years at the request of the incident commander is required to participate in the operation, to the extent that his or her skills, health and physical strength allows. Primarily, of course, volunteers are used. Anyone who, because of official duties or voluntarily, has been involved in an operation is entitled to reimbursement of travel and subsistence expenses, labour and loss of time, and compensation for damage to clothing and other personal belongings.

Conduct Surveillance at the Expense of Others

As mentioned previously, when the incident commander makes the decision to end an operation, the owner or tenant of the property should be notified that the operation has been ended and the need for security, salvage, restoration and recovery. If this is not possible and therefore not realised, and it is deemed necessary in view of the risk of a subsequent accident, the incident commander may provide security at the owner's or the right holder's expense.

Request Assistance of Other Authority

The incident commander may request any local, regional or national authority to participate in a fire and rescue operation. Such authorities are liable to contribute if the authority has the right capabilities and participation will not seriously hinder their normal operations.

Notify the Authority Responsible for Defects or Irregularities That Could Lead to Other Emergencies

If a deficiency or an anomaly that could lead to other emergencies or fire is encountered, the incident commander is obliged to inform the appropriate authority of the possibility. This may include anomalies such as health and safety issues, criminal activities or if environmental protection is needed.

Labour Management Rights and Health and Safety Responsibilities

An employer has a rather far-reaching right to precisely direct the work by employees. Provided that nothing specific has been agreed in this area, the employer, therefore, usually has the right to manage, distribute and otherwise organise the work and the workforce. Also, to determine more specifically what tasks an employee is required to do can be covered by the labour management rights. If an employee has different workplaces, which can be the case for firefighters during operations, the employer can also have the rights to decide on the geographical location/place at which the employee is required to work. However, the employee may to some extent restrict the employer's labour management rights. Consequently, a firefighter must do the tasks that come with the employment as a firefighter. But a firefighter can refuse to do a task if it, for example, is considered to be too dangerous or beyond the competency of the firefighter.

Health and safety responsibilities include an obligation to be active and take action by eliminating or reducing the risk of illness and accidents at work so that the working environment is good. An employer must allocate the tasks in the organisation in such a way that one or more managers, supervisors or other employees are tasked to ensure that risks at work are prevented, and a satisfactory working environment is achieved. The employer must ensure that those who receive these data are competent and have the powers and resources needed. The employer must also ensure that they have sufficient knowledge of the rules relevant to the work environment, physical, psychological and social conditions suggesting risks of illness and accidents, measures to prevent illness and accidents, and working conditions conducive to a satisfactory working environment (Arbetsmiljöverket 2012).

It is a responsibility of the senior management in an organisation to distribute tasks related to health and safety issues, in most cases, to officers in the organisation. These can in turn distribute such tasks, if they have such rights, to their respective managers. However, the senior management always has an obligation to regularly monitor the task allocation so that this works in practice and, if necessary, make any changes necessary.

Consequently, labour management rights as well as health and safety responsibilities have a large impact on the work during an operation. An officer can make decisions on what firefighters should do, but firefighters are entitled to refuse to fulfil tasks given. For many years, there has been a very strong focus on the incident commander. However, the obligations and responsibilities that come with the role of incident commander are much less important than labour management rights and health and safety responsibilities, which has a much larger impact on an operation.

Organisation, Command and Control

Some early work on firefighting tactics (including rescue) was done by Fredholm (1991). This work has largely affected the Swedish training of firefighters and fire officers and consequently fire and rescue operations. In short, it defines fire and rescue tactics as well as a number of general conditions of importance for the forming of tactics. These general conditions include the tactical problem, ideal, situation, coordination, structural basis, routines, skills and tacit knowledge, codes or practice, training opportunities and research. Fredholm suggested each of these areas to be developed.

The work by Fredholm was followed by work such as Cedergård and Wennström (1998), Svensson (2002) and Svensson et al. (2009). Consequently, there has been a surprisingly large amount of development on tactics in the Swedish Fire Service of which most has been implemented in the training of firefighters and fire officers and, thus, it has affected the fire service to a large extent. Also, although primarily focussing on the fire and rescue service, the work by Cedergård and Wennström (1998) has influenced a number of other local, regional and national authorities to develop similar approaches in their respective command systems.

The purpose of leadership and a command system as part of an operation is of course to be able to perform effective and safe operations. Unfortunately, there is too often a strong focus on the role of the incident commander. An incident commander is the fire chief of the fire service organisation or the person appointed by him or her (2003:778). From a management perspective, however, the role of the incident commander is subordinate. One can hardly expect that a single individual can be able to handle all the problems that arise in connection to an operation. Tasks and powers must therefore be divided between several different managers (officers) with apposite skills. An appropriately organised operation is important to carry out the work effectively, and it is important that all officers involved in an operation have been allocated their respective roles in advance, understand what is expected of them and what information is required and the responsibilities and liabilities connected to their roles.

The command and control structure in the Swedish Fire Service has to a large extent been influenced by the viable systems model (VSM) (Beer 1972), adapted and implemented by Cedergårdh and Wennström (1998) and further developed, adapted and implemented by Svensson et al. (2009). The viable system model (VSM) expresses a model for a viable system; any system organised in such a way as to meet the demands of surviving in a changing environment is a viable system. One of the prime features of systems that survive is that they are adaptable.

According to VSM, a viable system is composed of five interacting subsystems (Beer, ibid). Generally, Subsystems 1–3 are concerned with the 'here and now' of the organisation's operations, Subsystem 4 is concerned with the 'there and then', which are the strategic responses to the effects of external, environmental and future demands on the organisation. Subsystem 5 is concerned with balancing the 'here and now' and the 'there and then' to give policy directives which maintain the organisation as a viable entity. In addition to the subsystems, the environment is represented in the model. The presence of the environment in the model is necessary as the domain of action of the system. Without it, there is no way in the model to contextualise or ground the internal interactions of the organisation.

This was further developed, adapted and implemented by Svensson et al. (2009). According to this work, the management of fire and rescue operations should include:

- Foresight – long and short-term perspectives
  Command and control during operations must consider events, procedures and tasks in the long-terms as well as the short-term perspectives. It is not sufficient, which can often be the case, to consider ongoing events only.
- Flexibility
  Due to the inherent dynamics in operations, there must be a large degree of flexibility: the organisation and its staff must be able to adapt to changing conditions, conditions that change due to the nature of the event as well as due to procedures taken by the fire service.
- The need for assistance must be at the centre
  People call for help and they expect help, which must stay in focus throughout the operation. There is no end in itself to perform operations, there has to be a purpose, and objectives have to be set for each operation.
- Logic in roles
  There must be reasonable expectations placed on firefighters and fire officers, and they must have adequate education and training for the situations they approach.
- Risks, contingency and operations
  In addition to ongoing operations, the command system must also manage contingency as well as risks in the local community.
- Efficient use of resources
  Available resources should be used efficiently, including allocation of resources to wherever a need arises.
- Dynamic situation
  The command system must have an awareness of the inherent dynamics in operation: operations are like a game of chess where chess pieces as well as the game board changes character continuously.
- To gain and maintain control

To gain and maintain control can be said to be the overall objective of an operation.

- Leadership is important for individuals, groups and organisations
Fire and rescue operations are performed by individuals working in teams, and the command system must pay attention to how this affects operations.

Overall, the command and control system in the Swedish Fire and Rescue Service is considered to be a viable system, able to meet the demands of adapting in a changing environment. This is based on relatively well-trained and experienced firefighters and fire officers.

The command system is based on several parts, where the affected context describes and consists of those parts of society where a need for help arises due to an event, and the operational context describes and defines actors who should cooperate and coordinate their activities during response. In the command system used, three levels are identified: to execute tasks, to execute operations and to provide municipal fire and rescue service. To each of these levels, a decision domain is linked; system command, operation command and task command, which describes and defines a set of decisions that can be inflicted by the command level and thus affects its surroundings.

In the model, the decision domain task command is a subset of the decision domain operation command which in turn is a subset of the decision domain system command. The decision domain system command comprises all the other decision domains so that the model becomes a coherent system of interactions between the distributed decision-making, where system command is tied to the overall responsibility (Fig. 14.1).

The decision domain *system command* defines the role of the organisation, in relation to other organisations involved in the event; it defines the framework for operations (in terms of intentions of operations, resources, geography); it provides resources over time, and it manages preparedness in relation to the overall level of risk. This decision domain is the overall command function responsible for the fire service organisation.

The decision domain *operational command* determines objectives for an individual operation, decides and assigns tasks to units involved in the operation and coordinates the operation. In most cases, the role of an incident commander is linked to this decision domain. The domain is linked to a single operation and, consequently, there can be several such decision domains in case there are several ongoing operations.

The decision domain *task command* manages units in their execution of assigned tasks and coordinates the effort to fulfil those tasks. In most cases, there are several such decisions domains within a single operation.

In the fire service, the term 'unit' is used to define a set of resources with some specific capacity. This resource may consist of a single person or, which is more common, a vehicle with a set of tools (including pumps, ladders, hydraulic cutters, etc.) and a number of firefighters (Svensson et al. 2009). So, 'unit' refers to an organisational element consisting of one or several individuals using certain

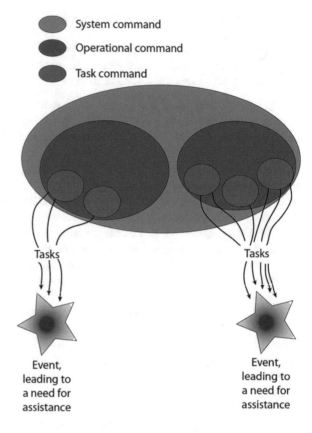

Fig. 14.1 Decision domains in the command system (Svensson et al. 2009)

equipment and certain skills having a certain ability to take action against all or part of one or more types of accident scenarios. The unit is assigned to one or more tasks and takes one or more actions to fulfil its task(s). The main purpose for creating units is to make resources easily manageable. From a management perspective, such a unit is the smallest part being handled. Units are usually defined in advance, but this does not exclude units being created or redefined during an ongoing operation based on the actual need.

One of the most common units within the Swedish Fire Service is known as a *base crew*, and it consists of a crew commander, four firefighters and a pumper/ fire truck. On such a truck, there are a variety of equipment, primarily for fighting fires and hydraulic equipment for the extrication of trapped people in car accidents. Also, this fire truck has equipment such as generators and lighting equipment as well as a variety of hand tools. This base crew unit is the basic unit in the fire and rescue service, and it can be expected to undertake a variety of assignments independently. It provides a very good opportunity for the crew to work effectively, whether it is a fire in a dustbin or a major disaster. The composition of the base crew is based on safety regulations for structural firefighting, as explained above (AFS 2007:7).

Other units in the fire service may be water units (tankers, water tenders), height units (ladders, platforms, snorkels, etc.), rescue units (cranes, trucks, etc.) and command units (everything from minibuses and vans to demountable tents and individual officers).

Staffing and Procedures

Unlike many other countries, where the fire and rescue service to a large extent can be based on voluntary participation (although there usually are some kind of financial compensation involved), in Sweden, we only have full-time staff and part-time staff. There are thus no actual volunteers in the Swedish Fire Services. However, in many municipalities, there are volunteer firefighters who get some training, equipment, facilities and possibly other types of compensation in return for their appearance at calls. These volunteers can be used only by request for official duties, which is a decision linked to incident commander only (see above).

There are approximately 15,000 firefighters and fire officers in Sweden, of which about 4000 are full-time firefighters, and the rest are part-time (retained) firefighters. Part-time firefighters have another primary employer other than the fire service. They are on duty every 3 or 4 weeks and then have to be in the vicinity of the fire station, so that they can turn out from the fire station within about 6 min after a call. Full-time firefighters and fire officers are on standby at a fire station and respond within approximately 90 s after a call. Part-time firefighters get their calls through pagers after which they travel to a fire station, get their equipment and respond to the accident site. Unfortunately, over the past few years, there has been increasing difficulties recruiting part-time firefighters.

Also, it should be noted that even if the training for part-time firefighters is shorter than for full-time firefighters, it is similar and they are expected by the public to perform similarly. During operations, there is not really any difference in approach, tactics, methodology or technique. Differences may exist due to differences in experience. However, there are part-time firefighters with far greater experience of operational work than what many full-time firefighters have.

That which is highly characteristic to the fire service is the ability to work in environments that few others can do, especially with regard to the need for speed and the risks that can often be associated with the situations they are in or conditions they are working under. Fire and rescue service staff are largely accustomed to working in dynamic situations where they must, on numerous occasions, exhibit a very high degree of flexibility. However, there are still safety regulations that must be met, many of them issued by the Swedish Work Environment Authority (www.av.se). Safety is of high priority in the Swedish Fire and Rescue Service.

References

Arbetsmiljöansvar och straffansvar. *Arbetsmiljöverket.* 2012.

Arbetsmiljöverket (Work Environment Authority). http://www.av.se. 2016-01-31.

Arbetsmiljöverkets föreskrifter om Rök- och kemdykning. AFS 2007:7. (In Swedish: Regulations on BA operations).

Beer, S. (1972). *Brain of the firm.* Harmondsworth: The Penguin Press.

Brandlag, 1974:80 (Fire law issued in 1974).

Cedergårdh, E., & Wennström, O. (1998). *Grunder för ledning, generella principer för ledning av kommunala räddningsinsatser.* Karlstad: Statens räddningsverk.

Civil protection act (2003:778) (In Swedish: Lagen om skydd mot olyckor).

Civil protection regulation (2003:789) (In Swedish: förordningen om skydd mot olyckor).

Clark, N. O. (1947). *A study of mechanically produced foam for combating petrol fires.* Department of Science and Industry Research. Chemistry Research Special Report No. 6. London: H.M.S.O.

Engström, J. (2011). *Handlingsprogram för skydd mot olyckor Höga Kusten – Ådalen.* Räddningstjänsten Höga Kusten – Ådalen.

Fredholm, L., & Göransson, A-L. (2006). (reds.). *Ledning av räddningsinsatser i det komplexa samhället.* Räddningsverket.

Fredholm, L. (1991). *The development of rescue tactics, analysis and proposed methods.* (FOA report C50089–5.3). Sundbyberg: National Defense Research Establishment, Department of Human Studies.

Handlingsprogram för skydd mot olyckor som kan leda till räddningsinsats för Räddningstjänsten Syd 2012–2015. Räddningstjänst Syd. 2011.

Hird, D., et al. (1954). The use of high and low pressure water sprays against fully developed room fires. *Fire Research Note 388/1954.* Fire Research Station.

Lag (2006:544) om kommuners och landstings åtgärder inför och vid extraordinära händelser i fredstid och höjd beredskap.

Lagar och ansvarsförhållanden i det svenska brandväsendets historia (P90–070/92). Räddningsverket (Swedish Rescue Services Agency, in Swedish). 1992.

Local government act (in Swedish: Kommunallag). 1991:900.

Luftfartsförordningen (In Swedish: Aviation Regulations), 1986:171.

Michal, O. (1993). *Brandsyn förr och nu.* Statens räddningsverk.

MSBFS 2012:5. *Myndigheten för samhällsskydd och beredskaps allmänna råd om ledning av insatser i kommunal räddningstjänst* (in Swedish: MSB regulations on command an control for the fire service when responding to accidents and incidents). Stockholm. 2012.

Räddningstjänst i samverkan (U30–666/08). Räddningsverket. 2008.

Shaw, E. M. (1876). *Fire protection, a complete manual of the organization, machinery, discipline, and general working of the fire brigade of London.* London: Charles and Edwin Layton.

Simms, D. L., & Hinkley, P. L. (1959). Protective clothing against flame and heat. *Fire Research Special Report No 3/1959.* Fire Research Station.

Statistics Sweden. Statistiska Centralbyrån. www.scb.se. 2016-01-31.

Svensson, S. (2002). *The Operational Problem of Fire Control* (doctoral thesis/report 1025). Lund University: Department of Fire Safety Engineering.

Svensson, S., Cedergårdh, E., Mårtensson, O., & Winnberg, T. (2009). *Tactics, command, leadership.* Karlstad: Swedish Civil Contingencies Agency.

The Swedish Civil Contingencies Agency. http://www.msb.se. 2016-01-31.

Thomas, P. H., & Smart, P. M. T. (1954). Fire extinction tests in rooms. *Fire Research Note 121/1954.* Fire Research Station.

Thomas, P. H. (1959). Use of water in the extinction of large fires. *The Institution of Fire Engineers Quarterly, 19*(35), 130–132.

Wargclou, D. (Ed.). (2010). *Räddningstjänst vid trafikolycka – personbil.* Myndigheten för samhällsskydd och beredskap.

Dr. Stefan Svensson   is an Associate Professor at Lund University, responsible for the fire laboratory and the experimental work at the Division of Fire Safety Engineering. Dr Svensson started his career as a firefighter in the Swedish Air Force in 1986. In 1989, he earned a bachelor's degree in fire safety engineering and, in 2002, a Ph.D. at Lund University, Sweden. Since 1994, he has been involved in experimental and theoretical investigations on firefighting tactics, including firefighting methods as well as problems of command and control. Educating firefighters, fire officers, postgraduates and Ph.D. students is and has been a large part of the work over the years, nationally as well as internationally. The safe and effective use of firefighting resources is a particularly important feature of his work, especially in relation to fire safety design of buildings. Also, he is the author of several books, scientific articles and reports. He is involved at the local fire brigade, as a firefighter/crew commander, and he has the rare ability to apply scientific knowledge in a very practical manner.

Chapter 15
2016 and the Future: Changing the Governance Paradigm as Well as the Operating Environment if Not the Financial Context

Peter Murphy and Kirsten Greenhalgh

As we approach the end of 2016 with the Crime and Policing Bill completing its parliamentary passage onto the statute book, it seems appropriate to be concluding this book with a look at what has happened in 2016 before briefly looking to the future and handing the analytic baton over to a future project.

In 2015, the UK had a general election which saw the return of a majority Conservative Government under the leadership of David Cameron. His short second administration continued with similar economic policies, and the same Chancellor of the Exchequer, George Osbourne, as had the previous coalition government. As with the coalition government, the economic strategy was dominated by policies of austerity and public sector spending restrictions. Even this, however, was overshadowed by a bigger debate over the UK's membership of the European Union (EU), as a result of the prime minister's promise in the election manifesto of a referendum on the country's continuing membership of the EU.

In May 2016, in what came to be seen as a pivotal and momentous event, the country voted in the referendum and, with a relatively small margin by the standards of national referendums, to leave the European Union. David Cameron who had campaigned to 'remain' resigned as the prime minister in June and as a member of parliament in September. He was replaced in July 2016 by his former Home Secretary Theresa May. Since being appointed in 2010, Theresa May had been one of the longest serving Home Secretaries in modern history. In her own view, she was responsible for a historical change in the nature of policing and had transformed the police services through a series of initiatives (Home Office 2016a, b, c).

She was also one of the three front runners for the leadership of the Conservative party alongside the Chancellor of the Exchequer, George Osbourne, and the former

P. Murphy (✉)
Nottingham Business School, Nottingham Trent University, Nottingham, UK
e-mail: Peter.Murphy@ntu.ac.uk

K. Greenhalgh
Nottingham University Business School, University of Nottingham, Nottingham, UK

© Springer International Publishing AG 2018
P. Murphy, K. Greenhalgh (eds.), *Fire and Rescue Services*,
DOI 10.1007/978-3-319-62155-5_15

Mayor of London, Boris Johnson. While the latter two spent much of 2015 and early 2016 as high-profile opponents on either side of the EU debate that was eventually to hamper them in the leadership contest, Mrs May discovered an extension to her policy agenda for police reform that had strong approval ratings within her own party and occasioned only muted opposition from the other political parties.

In 2012, Theresa May had introduced directly elected Police and Crime Commissioners (PCCs) which she subsequently perceived were politically popular across the major parties (Home Office 2015, 2016a, c, d). Despite a historically low turnout for the first elections of PCCs, the Conservative Manifesto for the 2015 had stated 'we will enable fire and police services to work more closely together and develop the role of our elected and accountable Police and Crime Commissioners' (Conservative Party 2015 p.59). They also proposed that in order generate greater engagement and democratic legitimacy, as a result of expected higher voting turnout, the second elections for PCCs should coincide with the local government elections in May 2016.

In September 2015, immediately after the summer recess, she therefore issued proposals through a consultation process (Home Office 2015) that was both extremely limited and much derided (Murphy 2015). By January 2016, largely ignoring the response to this consultation, she announced that the government intended to allow directly elected Police and Crime Commissioners to take over responsibility for Fire and Rescue Services (FRSs) 'where it is in the interests of economy, efficiency and effectiveness or public safety, and where a local case is made' (Her Majesty's Government 2016 p.10).

She was encouraged and empowered to do this, not only because of the weakness of the opposition and the distraction of the EU debate but also because the government had recently decided to transfer responsibility for the Fire and Rescue Services back to the Home Office, where responsibility for the police resides, from the Department of Communities and Local Government (DCLG).

This transfer of responsibility followed two excoriating reviews by the National Audit Office (NAO) of DCLG's previous oversight of Fire and Rescue Services over the previous 5 years (NAO 2015a, b). Although this transfer did not avoid the review of the NAO's reports by the Public Accounts Committee, who were equally scathing (Public Accounts Committee 2016), it enabled Mrs May in her last major speech as Home Secretary to announce that new amendments would be included at the committee stages of the 2016 Policing and Crime Bill to enable PCCs to take over Fire and Rescue Services and to facilitate joint working between the emergency services. There would also be improved consistency in fire standards, increased joint procurement of equipment and publicly available performance information. Ironically, all of these requirements resulted directly from the actions of the previous coalition government and were ongoing under previous labour administrations. She also committed the government to re-establishing an independent fire inspector (Home Office 2016d) which had effectively disappeared under labour in 2007.

Whether or not the provisions of the draft Policing and Crime Bill were carried over to the new parliament after the EU referendum and the summer recess became irrelevant, once Mrs May became the prime minister in July 2016. The Policing and Crime Bill was reintroduced in September 2016 and by November 2016 it had passed through all remaining stages in both Houses of Parliament. It received Royal Assent in January 2017 and the Policing and Crime Act (2017) came into effect on the 3rd April 2017.

During this time, the Fire Industry Association, the Fire Service College and the Chief Fire Officers Association began to collectively work with the government on new fire standards and procurement. The Home Office commissioned Her Majesty's Inspectorate of Constabulary to 'scope' and provide advice on the proposed new Inspectorate, and the Chief Fire Officers Association has revised its leadership and governance arrangements to enable the Association to play a more proactive role than has been the case since the 2004 Act.

Future Funding of the Service

On 23 November 2016, Philip Hammond presented his first budget to parliament as Chancellor of the Exchequer. This budget had three big fundamental elements that framed the rest of the budget. He announced revised growth targets for the future of the economy in 2017, a huge increase in government borrowing and more significantly but less obviously newsworthy, that there would be no changes to central government's Departmental Expenditure Limits (DEL), from those previously announced for the period 2015–2020. He also announced that these levels of expenditure would not be increased in line with inflation until after 2020/2021.

Members of the public are generally unfamiliar with the details or definitions of Departmental Expenditure Limits and announced in this way, they occasioned no headlines in any part of the media. However, DELs are the amounts of money that individual central government departments are allowed to spend. In practice, what the Chancellor said was that spending by the Home Office, like all the central spending departments, would be capped in cash terms and reduced in real terms for the remainder of the current electoral term up to 2020. The era of austerity in terms of limits on public expenditure was set to continue (House of Commons Library 2016).

Fire and Rescue Governance and Police and Crime Commissioners

The local leadership, governance and management of Fire and Rescue Services is likely to take a number of disparate forms as a result of the Policing and Crime Act. In London, where there is already an elected mayor, and in Manchester, the West Midlands, Merseyside, Tees Valley and Sheffield,[1] where there are anticipated to be elected mayors from 2017, the mayor will assume responsibility for Fire and Rescue Services as a result of the combined authority and devolution deals agreed under the Cities and Local Government Devolution Act 2016. However, as the new prime minister has indicated that elected mayors will not henceforth be a requisite for future combined authority deals, it is unlikely that many more elected mayors will be forthcoming (Sherman 2016).

Other areas will have the discretion to transfer Fire and Rescue Services to PCCs if a 'local case is made', or alternatively, PCCs can be invited to sit on the Fire and Rescue Authority (FRA). As this can happen in single authorities, combined authorities or metropolitan authorities, the range and type of governance arrangements in England and Wales will inevitably increase.

In Scotland and Northern Ireland, neither the Local Government Act 2000 nor the 2016 Cities and Local Government Devolution Act apply; both have single Fire and Rescue Services answerable directly to the devolved administration. In Wales, there are 4 police services and 4 PCCs, although there are 3 fire authorities – all 3 of which are 'combined' authorities. There are no directly elected mayors in Wales. Although the Cities and Local Government Devolution Act 2016 applies to Wales as well as to England, its practical effect is limited to potential changes in voting age that would take effect in Wales as well as in England if a change is made.

In England and Wales, there will be greater variety in the number and types of governance arrangements but it is still too early to predict the geographical pattern. As Chapter 13 has demonstrated, there is a single service in Scotland (Scottish Government 2016) which is coterminous with the ambulance service and the single police service. It has been operating well since it emerged from the amalgamation of the previous 8 services (Audit Scotland 2015). Scotland also has its own independent fire inspectorate and external regulation arrangements and it is therefore possible to foresee a more stable future in comparison with England and Wales.

The second direct elections for PCCs were held in 2016 in 40 areas (London and Greater Manchester were excluded because of the mayoralty situation). Table 15.1 shows the number of candidates standing and the political party representation. Both the number of candidates standing and the results (Table 15.2) show how the second election was dominated by the main political parties and the number of independent PCCs dropped from 12 to 3, all of whom were re-elections of previous PCCs. The Conservative and Labour parties shared the vast majority of successes while Plaid Cymru won 2 out of the 4 Welsh elections with Labour taking the other 2.

Twenty-seven of the existing 40 commissioners re-stood and 20 were elected. Thus, there were 20 new commissioners.

Despite the elections being held at the same time and in the same polling stations as the local government elections, the turnout averaged only 26% (previously 15%) and was noticeably higher where there was a local government election than when there was not, thus extending the argument about the political and democratic mandate and legitimacy attached to the post and the post holders.

The European Agenda

In the same month (November 2016) that the Policing and Crime Bill passed its parliamentary legislative process and the treasury announced the future funding plans, an international group of organisations with a common interest in Fire and

Table 15.1 Number of candidates standing in the 40 PCC elections in 2015

40	Conservatives
40	Labour
34	UKIP
30	Liberal Democrats
24	Independents
7	Greens
4	Paid Cymru (4 Welsh areas)
4	English Democrats
3	Zero Tolerance policing ex Chief

Table 15.2 Police and Crime Commissioners pre- and post-2015

	Pre-election	Post-election
Conservative	16	20
Labour	13	15
Independent	12	3
Plaid Cymru		2

Rescue Services, 'Fire Safe Europe',[2] called for the European Union to create a coordinated approach to fire safety in the EU. It claimed that the 'EU is working mostly in an indirect and uncoordinated manner, on a number of issues that could have an adverse effect on fire safety of buildings and occupants, yet fire safety is rarely a consideration when these policies are developed' (Fire Safe Europe 2016, p.7). It suggested that there is a patchwork of measures at national level and that the nature of fires had changed because more combustible materials are causing fires to grow more quickly than ever before. This is aggravated by the trend towards 'highly insulated airtight buildings with increased use of combustibles within the building envelope and structure' (2016, p4). At the same time:

- The EU is introducing directives and regulations that adversely affect fire safety in buildings.
- Fire-related building regulations are inconsistent from country to country across the EU.
- Construction product-testing protocols for fire safety are not continuously evaluated in relation to risks emerging from new construction trends as well as new threats, such as wildland fires. As a result, some are outdated. Regulation cannot be considered 'better' if it does not address the risks EU citizens may face.

Pointing out that fire safety is an issue that affects many policy areas, and that almost one-third of the European Commissions' Directorates Generals have disparate legislation that affects fire safety, it calls for better regulation and a European-wide strategy to ensure that new and renovated buildings across the EU are resilient to fires and that prevention programmes and policies are coordinated across member states.

Once again, it appears that Europe is set to address the variations, inconsistencies and challenges of improving fire safety while emphasising the distinctive nature and potential contribution of the service. Meanwhile, in England, the government is focussed on finance and governance and indirectly making it more difficult for the service to contribute to these sorts of international initiatives, further compromising the historical reputation for international leadership that has always been a characteristic of the UK services.

Notes

1. These are the areas that have taken part in 'Devolution Deals' with central government, although there are not absolutely certain as, at the time of writing, some are subject to legal challenge.
2. Fire Safe Europe is a collaboration between Brandfolkenes Cancerforening; Consumers safety International; CWB Fire Safety Ltd., European Fire Sprinkler Network; European Emergency Number Association; European Furniture Industries Confederation; European Organisation for Technical Assessment; Faculty of Civil Engineering, University of Zagreb; Federation de L'Industrie du Breton; Fire Service College; Fire Sector Federation; Centre for Technological Risk Studies; and Universitat Polictecnica de Catalunya.

References

Audit Scotland. (2015). *Scottish fire and rescue service*. Edinburgh: Audit Scotland.

Conservative Party. (2015). *The conservative party manifesto: Strong leadership, a clear economic plan, a brighter, more secure future*. London: The Conservative Party.

Fire Safe Europe. (2016). *Call to action: The EU needs a fire safety strategy.* Available at fire-safeeurope.eu/wp-content/uploads/2016/11/The-EU-needs-a-Fire-Safety-Strategy-1.pdf.

Her Majesty's Government. (2016). *Enabling closer working between the emergency services: Summary of consultation responses and next steps*. London: TSO.

Home Office. (2015). *Consultation: Enabling closer working between the emergency services.* London: TSO.

Home Office. (2016a). Home Secretary's speech Police and Crime Commissioners the choice is yours. 13th April 2016. Available at https://www.gov.uk/government/announcements?departments%5B%5D=home-office&page=3.

Home Office. (2016b). Home Secretary's Police Federation Conference 2016 Speech 17th May 2016. https://www.gov.uk/government/announcements?departments%5B%5D=home-office&page=3.

Home Office. (2016c). Home Secretary's speech to the Association of Police and Crime Commissioners 26th May 2016. https://www.gov.uk/government/announcements?departments%5B%5D=home-office&page=3.

Home Office. (2016d) Home Secretary speech on fire reform: Home Secretary Theresa May addresses audiennce at Reform event. 24th May 2016. Available at https://www.gov.uk/government/speeches/homeseretary-speech-on-fire-reform.

House of Commons Library. (2016) Fire service funding in England London House of Commons.

Murphy, P. (2015). Plans to merge fire and police services have dodged proper scrutiny. Putting police in charge of firefighters could lead to neglect of emergency services – Something the sham public consultation failed to mention. *The Guardian*. ISSN 0261-3077.

National Audit Office. (2015a). *Financial sustainability of fire and rescue services value for money report*. London: NAO.

National Audit Office. (2015b). *Financial sustainability of fire and rescue services local government report*. London: NAO.

Public Accounts Committee. (2016). *Financial sustainability of fire and rescue services*. London: House of Commons.

Scottish Government. (2016). *Fire and rescue framework for Scotland 2016*. Edinburgh: Scottish Government.

Sherman, J. (2016, August 22). May to abandon Osbourne's plan for regional mayors. *The Times*.

Index

© Springer International Publishing AG 2018   235
P. Murphy, K. Greenhalgh (eds.), *Fire and Rescue Services*,
DOI 10.1007/978-3-319-62155-5

Printed in the United States
By Bookmasters